Handbook of Urology

John James SRN
Charge Nurse, Urology/Surgical Unit
Broadgreen Hospital, Liverpool

Harper & Row, Publishers
London

Cambridge	San Francisco
Hagerstown	Mexico City
Philadelphia	Sao Paulo
New York	Sydney

First published 1984

Harper & Row
28 Tavistock Street
London WC2E 7PN

British Library Cataloguing in Publication Data

James, John,
A handbook of urology.1. Urinary organs — Diseases
I. Title
616.6 RC900

ISBN 0-06-318287-4

Typeset by Gedset Limited, Cheltenham.
Printed and bound by Butler & Tanner Ltd
Frome and London

CONTENTS

INTRODUCTION

This book commenced its life as a few brief guidelines kept on the ward explaining some of the more common urological conditions, operations, and techniques. For this reason some of the rarer conditions have been omitted. I have not included a detailed section on anatomy and physiology but have tried to put across some of the more specific knowledge and nursing skills I have gained during my work on a urological ward.

The chapters on infertility and incontinence contain reference to the work of a gynaecologist and much more detailed information on these techniques can be gained from specialized works. I have tried to keep it as straightforward as possible and hope both nurses in training and trained nurses coming to urology find this book of value.

JA JAMES
1984

ACKNOWLEDGEMENTS

I would like to thank all the people who gave me support and encouragement to take those first few notes and expand them into this text, in particular my wife for her invaluable help and love, and my parents for their support. Thanks must go to all the nursing staff past and present of B1 ward at Broadgreen Hospital especially Sister Ruth Graham and all the doctors with whom I have worked who offered constructive advice and gave invaluable assistance. Also Mr AD Desmond, Consultant Urologist, who gave me encouragement, and Mr J Gow who first fired my interest in urology.

Without the invaluable typing skills of Colette Nolan and the help of Sue Welch I don't think I would have ever completed this task. Finally thanks must go to Hilda Hodge, Broadgreen Hospital librarian, for her valued assistance, and Mr A Lyons, Nursing Officer, Surgical Unit, Broadgreen Hospital.

URINARY SIGNS AND SYMPTOMS

To pass urine — urination, voiding, micturition

Anuria   No urine production by the kidney (see retention of urine)

Azoospermia   No sperm in the semen

Bacteriuria   Bacteria in the urine

Clot retention   A complication of bleeding in the urinary tract

Cystitis   Inflammation of the bladder

Dysuria   Painful micturition, with difficulty

Enuresis   Incontinence of urine

Nocturnal enuresis Bedwetting at night

Frequency   Passing of urine very frequently

Glycosuria   Glucose in the urine

Haematuria   Blood in the urine

Hesitancy   Desire to pass urine but with delay in actual voiding

Nocturia   Voluntary passing of urine at night

Oligospermia   Abnormally low sperm numbers in semen

Oliguria   Diminished urine production by kidneys (less than 500 ml/24 hours)

Polyuria   Excessive production of urine (as in diabetes mellitus)

Proteinuria   Protein in the urine

Retention of urine   Inability to void, urine therefore accumulates in the bladder

Strangury   Painful straining to pass urine

Uraemia   Elevation of urea content of the blood

Urgency   Urgency to void

ANATOMICAL NOTES

The Urinary System (Fig.1)

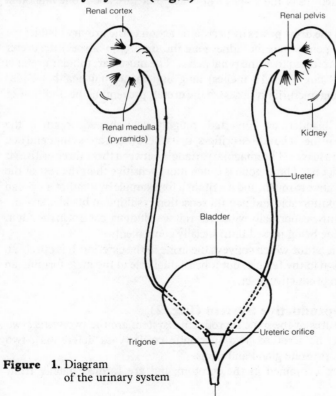

Renal cortex

Renal pelvis

Renal medulla
(pyramids)

Kidney

Ureter

Bladder

Ureteric orifice

Trigone

Figure 1. Diagram
of the urinary system

Urethra

The two kidneys, two ureters, the urinary bladder and the urethra form the urinary system. The kidneys have a characteristic shape and are about 10 cm (4 inches) long, 6 cm (2.5 inches) wide and 2.5 cm (1 inch) thick and are surrounded by fascia and fat. They lie behind the peritoneum adjacent to the upper lumbar vertebrae and 12th thoracic rib, and have an outer fibrous coat or capsule covering the renal tissue. The renal tissue has a distinctive appearance consisting of an outer brown coloured area of tissue or cortex, and an inner medulla which forms the renal pyramids. These renal pyramids project into the calyces (singular = calyx).

Supplied with blood directly from the renal artery, the renal vein empties directly into the inferior vena cava. The kidney's functions are to maintain the blood alkalinity, maintain body water balance, and excrete toxins and drugs. These are achieved during the production of urine by the nephrons (the microscopic structures of the kidney), of which there are about one million in each kidney.

Once formed the urine passes by peristaltic action to the urinary bladder via the ureter. At the point where the kidney joins the ureter (the calyces), the ureter is dilated, and is referred to as the renal pelvis. The muscular, tubular ureter is about 25.5 - 30 cm (10 - 12 inches) long and in normal health bladder contraction during micturition closes off the ureter, preventing the backflow of urine.

The urinary bladder, an inverted, roughly pear-shaped organ, is the reservoir for the urine. It has three orifices, two where the ureters enter and one where the urethra leaves. The imaginary triangle between these three orifices is known as the trigone. The trigone is much more sensitive than the rest of the bladder. It is sensitive to touch, and if irritated, for example by a catheter tip, can produce an uncomfortable and painful sensation resulting in bladder spasm.

A sphincter muscle, normally with over-riding voluntary control in the adult, prevents the urine being passed until socially convenient.

The urethra is a tube which conveys the urine to the exterior. It is purely an organ of excretion in the female, but it has a dual role in the male forming an element in the reproductive tract.

The Male Reproductive System (Fig. 2)

The main structures of the male reproductive system are the two testes, two epididymides in the scrotum, two spermatic cords (vasa deferentia), two seminal vesicles, prostate gland and penis.

The testes are contained in the scrotum and are formed mainly from

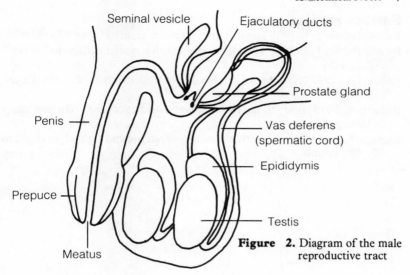

Figure 2. Diagram of the male reproductive tract

glandular tissue which produces the spermatozoa in tiny microscopic tubules. The testes also produce androgens, hormones responsible for the development of secondary sexual characteristics. Travelling via the epididymis and vas deferens (spermatic cord), the sperm reach the seminal vesicles, two small pouches near the bladder, which add secretions to the ejaculate and ejaculatory ducts.

The prostate gland lies just in front of the bladder and is normally about the size of a chestnut. The prostate lies around the urethra and it is easier to imagine it like an orange, the fleshy inner part (glandular tissue) surrounded by an outer peel (outer fibrous prostatic capsule). It is the fibrous capsule which acts as the urethra, following surgery to remove the prostate gland.

The urethra in the male is the pathway for both semen and urine and is much longer (15 - 18 cm; 6 - 7 inches) than the urethra in the female (2.5 cm; 1 inch). The urethra originates in the bladder at an internal sphincter muscle, passes through the prostatic region (prostatic urethra), to an external sphincter muscle. As it passes through the perineal region (membranous urethra), it bends markedly and finally reaches the outside at the meatus via the penile section.

The penis, composed of erectile tissue, surrounds the urethra; the skin covering the head of the penis is folded upon itself to form the foreskin or prepuce.

Further reading

Iveson-Iveson J (1979a) The urinary system, Nursing Mirror 148 (11): 31-32

Iveson-Iveson J (1979b) The male reproductive system, Nursing Mirror 148 (12): 33-34

Roberts A (1977) Systems of life No.25 Reproduction 1, Nursing Times 73 (1): supplt

Roberts A (1978) Body fluids 18: body water and its control, Nursing times 74 (47): supplt

Roberts A (1981) Reproductive system — systems and signs, Nursing Times 77 (49): supplt

CHAPTER 1

URINARY INVESTIGATIONS

Testing urine

1. Use a clean container for each fresh specimen.
2. Pay careful attention to technique — read instructions carefully, as failure to do so may not demonstrate an important abnormality.

The most commonly used testing agents are reagent dip and read sticks, such as Labstix or BN sticks, although specific tablets and strips are available, e.g. Acetest and Clinitest tablets. The dip and read strips are made of paper impregnated with chemicals which react to different substances. The strips must be kept dry when not in use. The paper must not be touched with the fingers as it may affect the result. Make sure the results are charted on the case sheet, nursing report, and/or urinalysis chart.

Colour

Urine is usually amber and transparent. In normal health, dark urine is concentrated; pale urine is dilute.

Drugs can affect the colour of urine, e.g. following lymphangiogram, urine turns blue/green, danthron (Dorbanex) turns urine red. Food also affects the colour of urine, e.g. eating beetroot can turn the urine red.

Other factors which should be considered are bile (bilirubin), urobilogen, lymph (kyleuria), which can also discolour/affect the general appearance of urine. Stale blood often gives urine a 'smoky' or dusky appearance. A fishy smell is characteristic of urinary infection.

Amount

The average amount of urine passed 1500 ml/24 hours. Causes of abnormal volume include:

1. Polyuria — diabetes insipidus, uncontrolled diabetes mellitus.
2. Dysuria — acute pylonephritis, dehydration, urethritis.
3. Anuria — acute nephritis, malignant pelvic growth, crush injury, incompatible infusion, shock (low blood pressure), acute renal tubular necrosis.
4. Urinary retention — prostatic enlargement.

Reaction

Urine is usually acid, i.e. pH6, pH5 (pH7 is neutral). Alkaline urine, i.e. pH8, pH9, indicates a stale specimen, sodium bicarbonate or potassium citrate therapy, urine tract infection.

Specific gravity

Specific gravity is measured with a urinometer, (hydrometer) (Fig.3). An early morning specimen is the most concentrated; normal range is 1015 — 1025.

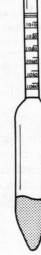

Figure 3. Diagram to show a
urinometer used for the
measurement of urine
specific gravity

1. Increased — concentrated urine indicates glycosuria, e.g. diabetes mellitus, dehydration.

2. Decreased — dilute urine indicates decreased kidney efficiency, diabetes insipidus, over drinking, diuretic drugs.

Urine osmolality is a more elaborate test for urine concentration.

Protein (albumen)

A positive reaction to protein may appear in infection but may also be significant of renal disease including nephrotic syndrome and glomerulonephritis. A false positive can be seen if reagent sticks are used incorrectly, e.g. timing wrongly before reading.

Sugar

Positive reactions to sugar appear in diabetes mellitus but a low kidney threshold to sugar will also cause this reaction even though the blood level is normal. Blood tests will determine this.

Ketones

A positive reaction is obtained when fat is not metabolized correctly, e.g. in diabetes mellitus. Acetest tablets also test for this.

Haematuria

Haematuria may appear in cases of malignancy, infection, trauma and stones. It may be visible to the naked eye (macroscopic), or only detectable on testing (microscopic). Macroscopic haematuria can be helpful in diagnosis. Bright red urine is suggestive of recent bleeding (any clots are usually jelly-like), while small black clots resembling tea leaves are suggestive of old bleeding. Blood cause discomfort on voiding, and large clots can cause retention of urine whether there is a catheter present or not.

Bacteriology of urine

Bacteriological tests of the urine are examinations of urine culture to identify micro-organisms in the patient's urine specimens. The laboratory uses the specimen for microscopic and chemical examinations. It is important when collecting urine specimens that:

1. An aseptic technique is employed to avoid contamination of specimens.

2. The container is sterile.

3. Care is taken to avoid contaminating the specimen. It should be exposed for the least possible time before being bottled. The specimen pot should be firmly closed with a screw cap so there is no fear of contamination of the urine on the way to the laboratory.

4. In taking speciments no harm should come to the patient. Catheter specimens should be taken by withdrawal of urine, using a needle and syringe from the specimen port. The catheter should not be disconnected from the drainage bag, as this increases the danger of introducing infection.

5. The specimen is labelled clearly and correctly. It is no use labelling a catheter specimen (CSU) as an MSSU (midstream specimen of urine) — they are different and should be labelled so.

6. Specimens are sent to the laboratory as soon as possible, as some micro-organisms die rapidly if the specimen is left to stand.

7. Urine taken at night or at the weekend should be kept refrigerated.

8. Specimens should be sent to the laboratory as early as possible in the day.

MSSU (midstream specimen of urine) collection

Urine passed in the normal way is usually contaminated by flora from around the meatus and for cultural examination midstream specimens are required. Specimens should be collected in the following manner:

1. The procedure is explained and the patient reassured that it is painless.

2. In the male patient — the prepuce is retracted, and the glans is washed.

3. In the female patient — the vulva is cleaned with sterile water or saline, although soap and water cleansing or a mild antiseptic solution is sometimes employed.

Many organisms are usually washed from the meatus in the initial streams of urine. Following the passing of the initial stream, the specimen is collected from the next 50 ml of urine and the remainder allowed to run away. In children specimen-taking is usually more difficult, and special collection bags are used. In infants urine can be aspirated by passing a fine needle through the abdomen into the bladder (suprapubic aspiration).

Urgent bacteriological tests can be carried out by the nurse using agar-impregnated dip sticks.

Ideally a midstream specimen should be collected prior to the commencement of antibiotic therapy.

Because of the high percentage of patients routinely admitted to surgical and urological wards, it is commonsense to make cultural specimens a routine admission procedure so that none get overlooked.

24-hour urine collection

This is the collection of the total urine passed in a 24-hour period. This is a painless procedure. However, care must be taken with the collection bottle as it sometimes contains a preservative which is corrosive.

The patient empties the bladder and this urine is discarded. It is important to note the time accurately and correctly. Each subsequent specimen of urine passed is collected in the container provided by the laboratory. During the test the patient can eat and drink normally. Some surgeons prefer the test to be taken when the patient is in his/her home environment, as results may vary with alterations in diet.

Twentyfour hours later, the patient empties the bladder, even if there is perhaps no obvious desire to void, and this urine is added to the collection. This completes the test and the urine is sent to the laboratory.

Twentyfour-hour urine collection is of value in the diagnosis of many conditions, including renal function tests, hormone gland studies, and renal calculi.

Cystometrogram (cystometry)

The bladder is the reservoir for urine and is usually emptied when socially convenient. If this voluntary neurogenic mechanism is upset (i.e. incontinence), it can be investigated by inserting a fine catheter into the bladder. By running in fluid, the pressure within the bladder increases and its effect can be recorded on a special graph. This can help in the diagnosis and further management of various conditions. This investigation demonstrates the following:

1. Awareness and response to filling.
2. When a senation to void is felt.
3. When voiding is compulsory.
4. The maximum volume the bladder can contain.
5. The stability of the bladder muscle.

These can all be compared with normal readings. The cystometrogram can also record the rate of the urine.

The surgeon can use flow rate measurement in the assessment of many conditions including urethral strictures, pre- and postoperative prostatic and bladder surgery, neurogenic disease.

To achieve a good overall picture, it is important that the patient voids at least 150 ml at the time of the examination. The date, patient's name, amount voided, and graph paper calibration are entered on the final recording.

Fluid balance

Maintaining an accurate record of a patient's fluid intake and output over 24 hours is vital to the urological management. These charts, when totalled, give a comparison between intake and output and, if accurately maintained, can demonstrate a positive or negative fluid balance. In illness the balance can be drastically disturbed and need urgent restoration. Fluid balance maintenance can make care less difficult and less dangerous.

Cystoscopy: urethroscopy (Fig. 4)

Cystoscopy is an examination of the lining of the bladder and the urethra using a long telescope fitted with a light for improved vision. It is the most important special method of investigation in urology. It is used in diagnosis of many conditions, e.g. haematuria, chronic urinary tract infection, and contraindicated in only a very few cases, e.g. acute urinary tract infection.

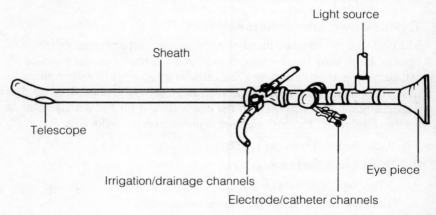

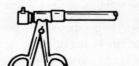

Figure 4. a. Diagram of a cystoscope.
         b. With biopsy forceps passed down

A cystoscope is a special piece of optical equipment. It consists of a telescope containing a lens mechanism which transmits the image of the bladder, urethra, ureteric orifice, etc., to the eye of the viewer. It is contained in a sheath, which is a round/oval metal catheter just large enough to accommodate the telescope. The sheath also has a small passage along its length for the light to be shone, (either by bulb or fibrelight, a plastic-coated cable containing glass fibres). A fibrelight cable should not be bent acutely as this can break some of the glass fibres, and reduce the light transmission.

A cystoscope is a very expensive and delicate instrument. To avoid damage to the lenses the telescope part is not used in the actual passage of the instrument but a metal obturator is inserted in its place. Biopsies may be taken by means of a pair of biopsy forceps passed down the sheath. Modern cystoscopes also have irrigation/drainage channels, to allow blood to be washed away when investigating haematuria, and as the bladder normally has many folds the fluid allows the entire bladder to be viewed. There is usually the facility, via further small channels in the sheath, to allow electrodes or catheters to be passed.

Cystoscopy may be performed under local epidural or general anaesthetic and patient preparation is minimal, e.g. fasting as routine before a general anaesthetic and following ward routine postoperatively.

Postoperative care consists of simple observations. The patient should be informed that some discomfort can be expected. Ensure that the patient micturates and that the urine is not heavily bloodstained, especially if the patient is being treated as a day case prior to discharge.

After epidural anaesthesia, the patient's legs will feel numb, so he must remain on bedrest, and must use a urine bottle in bed. The patient is admitted for a 24-hour, overnight stay. In some hospitals the tip of the removed epidural cannula is attached into the case sheets to demonstrate that the full cannula has been removed (for medico-legal reasons).

Radiological procedures

Intravenous pyelogram/urogram

An intravenous pyelogram (IVP) or intravenous urogram (IVU) is a radiological procedure, in which a fluid highlighted under x-ray (contrast medium) is injected into a vein, observed by image intensifier and photographed as it is excreted through the kidney (pyelogram), and through the rest of the urinary tract (urogram).

Patient preparation varies from department to department, but in general fluids are not taken for at least four hours before the procedure, and a laxative or enema is given prior to the x-ray. This is to avoid bowel content or gas obscuring the pictures of the urinary tract.

Allergic reaction to the iodine-containing contrast medium is not unknown and the radiologist should be informed of any history of asthma, hay fever, eczema or severe hypertension.

A small number of patients have a sensation of flushing or sickness following injection of the contrast medium. Some departments prefer the patients to wear a light gown to avoid problems with buttons or other x-ray opaque material affecting the film.

A film may be taken when the patient has passed urine at the end of the procedure to check that the bladder is empty or if there is any residual urine.

On completion of the x-ray, the patient will probably welcome a drink and something to eat, having been on a limited oral intake for some time.

Retrograde pyelogram

Retrograde pyelogram may be done following intravenous pyelogram/urogram if any of the following are demonstrated:

1. Poorly or non-functioning kidney.
2. Calculi.
3. Tumour.
4. Urethral stricture.
5. Inconclusive diagnosis.

The procedure is generally performed following cystoscopy under general anaesthetic. A small catheter is passed up the ureter, the scope is withdrawn, leaving the catheter in situ. Dye (contrast medium) is then passed up the catheter to outline the renal tract. Patient preparation is the same as for routine general anaesthetic with usual postoperative care.

Cysto-urethrogram (cystogram)

Cysto-urethrogram is usually performed on patients with a faulty mechanism in passing urine, e.g. stress incontinence or narrowed urethra. A catheter is inserted and contrast medium introduced. The patient is then x-rayed:

1. At rest.
2. Straining down without passing the fluid.
3. With the catheter out as the fluid is passed (micturating cystogram). A

x-ray can be used to see if there is a reflux up the ureter during urination (possible cause of chronic pyelonephritis).

Renal arteriography

Renal arteriography is an x-ray examination usually performed under general anaesthetic, to outline the renal blood supply. A fine catheter is passed up the femoral artery and aorta or is passed via the lumbar aorta to the renal artery where dye is injected. Renal arteriography is used mainly to differentiate renal masses, e.g. tumours and cysts. Following this procedure the patient remains on 24 hours bed rest. Careful observation of puncture site and blood pressure are essential as a major artery is punctured during the procedure.

Ultrasound scan

A permanent photographic record can be obtained of an organ's surface using high frequency sound waves. A water-soluble contact jelly is placed on the skin surface to prevent gas/air distorting the picture, then the high frequency sound waves are passed through the body and the reflected image recorded on a special recorder. This is used in urology to investigate kidney lesions and to monitor the extent of bladder tumours.

Preparation for ultrasound kidney scan tends to vary according to local policy, e.g. the patient may be fasted and a bowel evacuation performed. For ultrasound of the bladder a full bladder is required. The patient is therefore requested to drink three to four glasses of fluid (550-650 ml) one hour before examination. If the patient has a catheter in situ this is clamped at the same time. Rectal ultrasound probes are now available for examination of the prostate.

Lymphangiography

In lymphangiography x-rays are used to show lymphatic vessels and glands. It is used mainly to assess the spread of tumours (mostly testicular). A blue dye is injected between the toes, and is absorbed by the lymph vessels, which are then injected with contrast medium following a cut down procedure. No special patient preparation is needed except to remove hair from the feet. Patients should be warned that this is a long procedure, and may produce a bluish skin tinge and colour the urine blue/green when excreted.

Vasogram

Contrast medium is injected into the vas deferens to outline the spermatic cord in investigating male infertility.

Bone scan/renal scan

Bone/renal scan is sometimes used in determining the spread of a tumour. A low dose of radioactive substance is injected and taken up by the bones. This is observed and recorded by special equipment. The isotope used is also excreted via the kidney and so in the urological patient a picture of the kidneys may be obtained if there is any renal disease known or suspected. Patient preparation is usually minimal, but the reassurance of the patient regarding the low level of radioactive material employed is advisable.

Further reading

Ashby P R (1976) Refresher course — haematuria, Nursing Times 72 (9): 336

Elliot B A (1908) Urinalysis, Nursing (18): 784-786

Fay J (1979) Urine testing (and collection of specimens for culture), Nursing Mirror 149 (4): supplt

Hatcher J (1976) Quackery, fraud and scientific method, the history of urine testing, Nursing Mirror 142 (17): 65-66

Parfrey P S (1982) Proteinuria, British Journal of Hospital Medicine 27 (3):254-258

Smith T C G (1976) Specimen testing, Nursing Mirror 124 (22): 60-61

Weir T and Abrahams P (1980) X-ray anatomy 5 (IVP Retrograde Pyelogram, Renal Arteriograms), Nursing Times 76 (39): supplt

Weir T and Abrahams P (1976) X-rays in focus — post basic, Nursing Times 72 (36): supplt

CHAPTER 2

URETHRAL CATHETERS AND CATHETERIZATION

If the bladder is full and urine has not been passed for some time, the obvious discomfort the patient suffers demands some form of treatment. Measures other than catheterization which may help a patient to void include:

1. Giving the patient a warm bath;
2. Analgesia to allay pain/anxiety especially postoperatively;
3. Allowing the patient to stand beside the bed to use a urine bottle or to use the toilet;
4. Warming the bottle or bed pan;
5. The sound of running water;
6. Injection of distigmine bromide (Ubretid), 500 micrograms intramuscular. This drug stimulates bladder activity and is only used if the patient has non-obstructive retention of urine.

If these measures fail, catheterization may be required. This is a well-established procedure used for many years; records show its use in 3000 BC. Originally made of metal (bronze, silver and tin), catheters are now usually made of latex rubber, plastic or silicone. Modern catheters are normally individually packed and sterilized by gamma radiation.

The length of the catheter is important. There are shorter length catheters for use in female patients or in ambulant patients. The length of the catheter, however, does not alter the sizing, which is normally measured on the Charrière scale, which measures the circumference of the catheter in millimetres. The size is normally indicated by the number (size), and letters ch or fg written on the packet and the catheter itself, e.g. 16fg or 18ch. Catheters are often colour-coded to denote Charrière size. Most modern catheters in use are self-retaining,

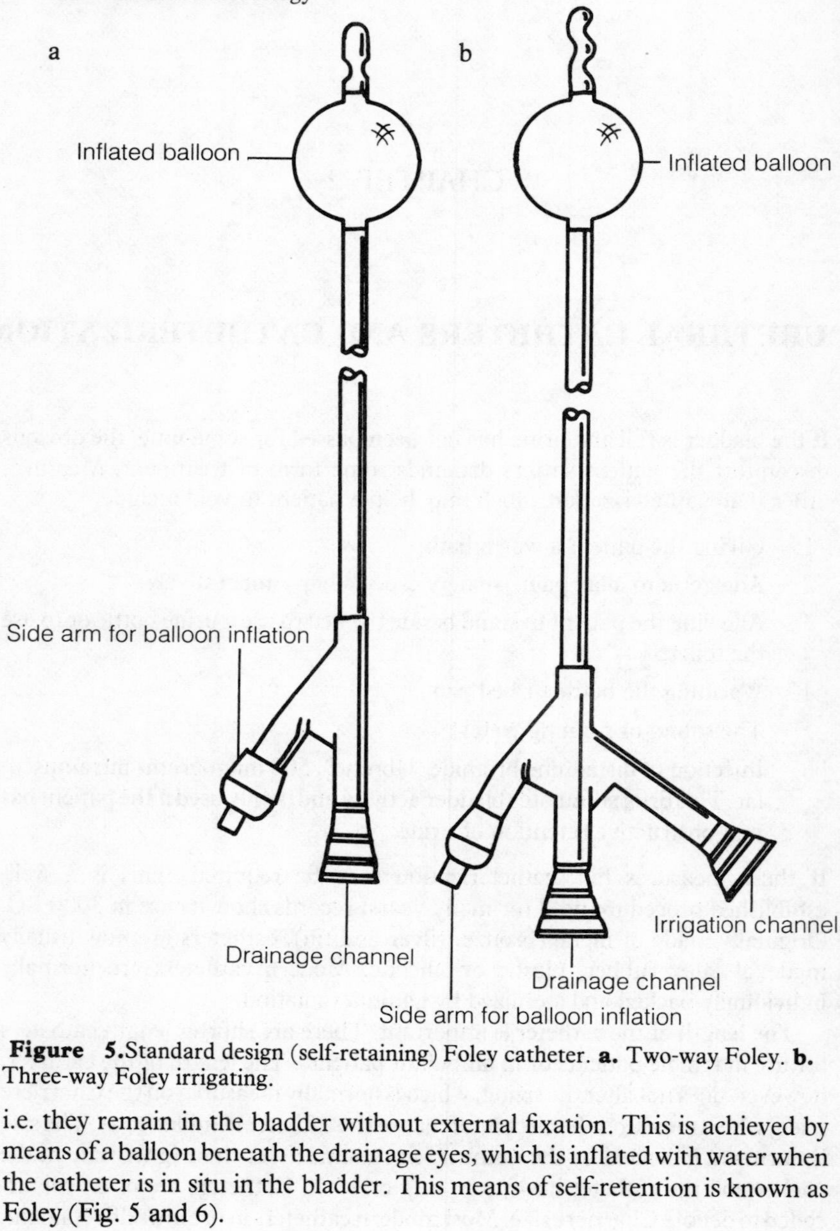

Figure 5. Standard design (self-retaining) Foley catheter. **a.** Two-way Foley. **b.** Three-way Foley irrigating.

i.e. they remain in the bladder without external fixation. This is achieved by means of a balloon beneath the drainage eyes, which is inflated with water when the catheter is in situ in the bladder. This means of self-retention is known as Foley (Fig. 5 and 6).

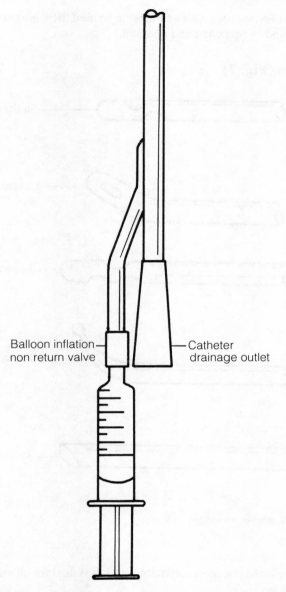

Balloon inflation non return valve

Catheter drainage outlet

Figure 6. Retention of catheter — inflation of the balloon with water and syringe

When considering the urinary catheter to be used there are two main points to bear in mind — tip design and material.

Tip design (Fig. 7)

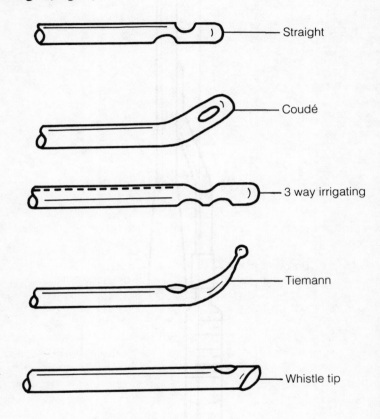

Figure 7. Catheter tip shapes

Straight
This catheter is the one most commonly used. It is used for all uncomplicated catheterizations.

Tiemann

These are used for ease of insertion in gross prostatic enlargement, but should only be used by experienced practitioners.

Coudé

This catheter is also used in cases of prostatic enlargement to enhance passage.

Whistle tip

These catheters are indicated for drainage of large clots, or where large amounts of debris are present. Some surgeons employ a whistle tip on a 3-way irrigation simplastic catheter in the management of postoperative urological patients, because the firm material does not collapse under negative pressure if washout/aspiration is performed.

Irrigation tip

This catheter has an eye to allow irrigation fluid to outflow and eyes to help free outflow/drainage.

Most catheters have drainage eyes above the Foley balloon. The Robert's catheter has drainage holes above and below the balloon to enhance complete bladder drainage. These are rather less commonly used at present.

Material construction

Latex

These inexpensive soft, rubber catheters are generally well tolerated by the patient, and are suitable for short term use (up to two weeks). They should be avoided in long term use (up to 12 weeks), as they tend to have thick walls with a fairly small drainage channel. They can occlude due to high debris formation around the catheter tip and balloon. They are rather difficult to pass in male patients with some prostatic enlargement, because of the softer material.

Plastic (simplastic)

Plastic catheters are also inexpensive, are stiffer than the latex rubber type and therefore tend to be easier to pass in cases of prostatic enlargement. They have thin walls which give the catheter good drainage and rarely become blocked. They seem to cause discomfort or rejection in long term use (12 weeks) due to balloon encrustation. They are more suitable in short term cases (2 weeks). An advantage is that they withstand aspiration to remove blockage and thus avoid having to change the catheter.

Silicone-coated latex rubber

Silicone-coated latex rubber catheters are well accepted and their construction reduces debris deposition. They have rather thick walls with correspondingly narrower channels, but this does not seem to affect their performance. They are ideally suited to long term use (12 weeks). Their higher cost tends to limit their short term use.

Some surgeons prefer to use teflon-coated catheters e.g. Barco — an inert material employed to reduce the possibility of irritation of the urethral lining, and to aid in the reduction of deposition of debris.

Solid (100%) silicone

Solid silicone catheters, though generally the most expensive, have the advantage of causing the least tissue reaction. In long term use (12 weeks) they produce few side effects, resisting encrustation well, and their wider bore tubing allows good drainage. They are often the catheter of choice in long term management, as they also produce little urethritis. They are well suited for use postoperatively, and are frequently used in the care after surgery of the urethra.

Gibbon catheters (Fig. 8)

Gibbon catheters are semi-rigid plastic catheters which are used rather less frequently than previously. The catheter is fixed externally by means of two plastic strips taped to the penis. They are used primarily for long term care to avoid Foley fixation problems, e.g. encrustation. Many doctors still prefer this type of catheter as they feel its plastic construction and small calibre, from 8fg upward, make it easy and fairly safe to pass. Its size reduces the likelihood of urethritis but its long term use does not allow the effective use of antiseptic bladder washouts which some urologists prefer.

Suprapubic catheters (sometimes called 'suprapubic cystotomy')

If there is obstruction of the urethra, urethral false passage, urethral stricture, or gross enlargement of the prostate, preoperative urethral catheterization may be difficult or dangerous. By inserting a drainage tube through the skin into the bladder in the suprapubic region, urine can be drained.

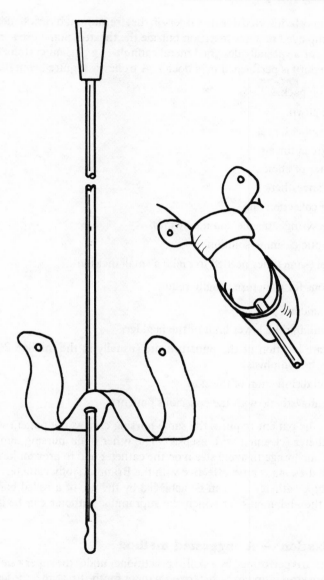

Figure 8.a Diagram of a Gibbon catheter. **b.** Gibbon catheter secured with tape in male patient

The tube may be inserted during surgery in theatre, although various designs have been employed to allow insertion outside the theatre. Some use a trocar (e.g. Argyle), or a specially designed metal cannula (e.g. Braun cystofix).

The procedure is performed by a doctor. A trolley is required containing:

1. Dressing pack.
2. Sterile gown.
3. Sterile gloves.
4. Two green towels.
5. Catheter of choice.
6. Local anaesthetic.
7. Sterile collection bag.
8. Sterile syringe, needle and mediwipes.
9. Antiseptic cleaning solution.
10. Scalpel (sometimes needed to make a small incision).

The conditions for puncture usually require:

1. Full bladder.
2. Determining the lower limit of the bladder.
3. Accurate location of the puncture site (usually in the midline 2-3 cm above the symphisis).
4. Careful disinfection of the skin.
5. Local anaesthetic with the conscious patient.

Once in situ the patient requires the same nursing care as the patient with a urethral catheter (cleaning with asepsis). The other main nursing aim is to afford good anchorage to avoid strain on the catheter and to prevent kinking. Op Site type dressing is most effective with the Braun cystofix catheter. With the Argyle type catheter this can be achieved by the use of a rolled bandage secured on the abdomen over which the suprapubic catheter can be gently curved.

Catheterization — A suggested method

Catheterization is performed by a skilled practitioner under the supervision of a doctor. Before attempting to catheterize a patient for the first time, the learner must have adequate demonstration and supervision in the clinical area.

The choice of catheter size is largely a matter of experience, but as a rough guide, in the adult a 12fg, 14fg or 16fg catheter should be adequate. If the urine is cloudy or bloodstained, an 18fg or 20fg may be chosen and only in cases of thick blood or pus being passed are 22fg or 24fg catheters required. These are only passed by very experienced practitioners.

In general the softest, narrowest catheter necessary to give effective drainage is selected. It must not be so large as to obstruct the para-urethral glands or restrict their secretions.

The Foley balloon generally come in two sizes — 5-10 ml and 15-30 ml. The smaller size is usually adequate as it tends to cause less bladder irritation in retaining the catheter. The larger balloon is used mainly in postoperative management, to ensure catheter retention when the bladder exit has been involved in surgery.

When catheterizing a male patient, some people like to use a penile clamp to retain the lignocaine gel and ensure adequate analgesia. Good lighting is a priority in catheterizing all patients, but especially in women who are somewhat overweight or elderly, as the urethra is often difficult to see. An anglepoise lamp can be most helpful and it is sometimes easier, if it is at all possible, to pass a catheter in these patients in a treatment room where they can lie on a firm couch with their legs supported. A gentle, slow technique is often the best approach. If the patient is worried, the bladder muscle tightens, and passing the catheter becomes difficult. Force must never be used as there is a risk of tearing the delicate urethral lining. If difficulty is encountered, medical help should be sought immediately.

Two people are required, one to perform the procedure and one to assist. A trolley is prepared containing:

1. Sterile gloves
2. Sterile gown
3. Catheter pack with two towels (a circumcision towel if available helps in the prevention of skin contamination
4. Catheter
5. Sterile 20 ml syringe
6. Sterile water (sufficient to inflate the balloon)
7. Sterile collection bag
8. Lignocaine gel

9.   Antiseptic cleaning solution.

The procedure is fully explained to the patient, and privacy ensured. Explanation of the procedure and telling the patient what to expect helps in the future management, e.g. in reducing infection, trauma and undue catheter movement. The pubic area is washed with soap and water and dried thoroughly.

The nurse washes and dries her hands and puts on the sterile gown. The trolley is taken to bedside, the catheter pack opened and the contents laid out; other packets are opened by the assistant — syringe and water to inflate the balloon, lignocaine gel and antiseptic solution.

The assistant prepares the patient, and arranges the top bed clothes. If possible the assistant places the patient in recumbent position with legs separated. The patient is asked to relax.

Male catheterization

A sterile towel is placed to cover the legs and scrotum and a second towel placed to cover the abdomen, exposing the penis only. A circumcision towel is used if one is available. The penis is not touched by hand. A piece of gauze is opened and folded in half, then placed around the penis. Only the gauze is held. The meatus is cleaned using cotton wool or preferably gauze swabs and antiseptic solution. Lignocaine gel is inserted into the urethra (using the application nozzle) and milked along the length of the penis. The use of a gel combined with an antiseptic (e.g. chlorhexidine) has obvious advantages in infection control. The nurse's hands are washed again and/or cleaned with antiseptic hand rub, e.g. Hibisol.

Only now are the catheter, sterile collection bag, and gloves opened. Some kits are available with the catheter already attached to the drainage bag. This ensures that the gloves are exposed for the briefest time possible before the catheter insertion.

Gloves are now applied, and the catheter inner wrap is removed or split to allow the catheter to be connected to the collection bag. This procedure ensures that the sterile catheter is only handled by a sterile gloved hand. The time taken for this procedure allows the lignocaine gel to become effective. The catheter is passed with the gloved hand or forceps while the gauze is held around the penis.

The penis is usually held at a right angle to the abdomen and the catheter introduced into the urethra. The external orifice (meatus) is the narrowest part of the urethra, so a catheter passing comfortably through this should pass easily down the rest of the urethra.

The catheter should be inserted gently and as it passes through the perineal region it has to be negotiated around a bend. As the catheter reaches this point it should be manoeuvred slowly while the penis is lowered toward the thighs. Once through this region the catheter reaches the prostatic area where the passage bends again. Difficulty may be encountered here and it is important that the patient does not tighten the bladder muscle, or that undue force is applied. As the catheter enters the bladder, urine should be seen to flow into the urine drainage bag.

The balloon should be inflated when free urine flow is clearly seen. If a catheter specimen of urine (CSU) is required, the first specimen may be taken from the collection bag, provided that the procedure has not been concluded, i.e. asepsis discontinued.

If the catheter is not to be retained, the balloon is not inflated, the catheter is removed and discarded. The patient is made comfortable, and the equipment is disposed of as for a dressing.

Female catheterization

The same basic procedure is followed and gauze swabs are used to part the vulva. The urethral opening lies anterior to the vagina within the labia.

Catheter management

Catheters are passed in different conditions including:

1. Enlarged prostate.
2. Urethral stricture.
3. Postoperative management.
4. Urethral or vesical calculi.
5. Injury or disease of spinal cord.
6. Ruptured urethra.
7. Blood clot retention (haematuria).
8. For accurate measurement of urine in severe illness, e.g. patients in intensive care.

In certain cases the surgeon may order short term catheterization. In urinary retention following surgery, a catheter is sometimes passed and then removed once the retention is relieved. It may be left in situ until the following morning if the patient is having a rather slower general postoperative recovery.

The need for a catheter should be assessed every day and it should be removed as soon as possible. It is better to avoid catheterizing on a long term basis if possible; alternatives may be considered, including incontinence aids e.g. penile sheaths (see incontinence), or intermittent catheterization e.g. in patients with spinal injuries.

In certain circumstances where the bladder needs stimulation, phenoxybenzamine 10 mg twice daily orally may be prescribed for 24 hours before catheter removal. This drug has been shown to reduce urinary outflow obstruction, possibly by relaxing nervous control of the bladder neck muscles. Care is taken in the administration of this drug in patients with hypotension (low blood pressure) as it can cause a fall in blood pressure when the patient is standing (postural hypotension). This drug is also associated with nasal stuffiness.

Urinary infection
Urinary tract infection can quickly follow catheterization. To minimize this;

1. Closed drainage is employed.
2. Open drainage is avoided.
3. Catheters are left alone when working well.
4. Catheter care is employed.

Closed drainage Closed drainage is used to reduce the routes and sources of infection. Once the catheter is in situ with drainage bag, it is not disturbed. Only drainage taps are employed to empty the bag and they must not be allowed to touch the floor. A non-return valve is used in the drainage bag. The connection between the catheter and drainage bag is not broken. Any attendant to the catheter wears clean gloves. However, the closed system does have external entry points for bacteria:

1. At the meatus between catheter and urethra.
2. The connection between the catheter and the urine bag.
3. The urine sampling port.
4. At the outlet drainage tap.

The non-return valve at the connection of the tube to the bag is aimed at reducing infection tracking upward. Infection control measures are generally employed when dealing with catheters to try to minimize infection at these points. One simple action to prevent urine reflux is to ensure that the bag is always below the level of the bladder e.g. avoid pinning the bag at waist level in mobile patients or putting the bag on their lap when they are in a chair or wheel chair.

Open drainage Open drainage greatly increases the infection risk. Open drainage consists of closing off the catheter with a spigot with intermittent release. It is not therefore good practice to retrain the bladder using this method; its risks are great and its effectiveness is suspect.

Recatheterizing the patient Recatheterizing the patient should be kept to a minimum, although certain units have the policy of regularly changing catheters even in the absence of manifest problems. The choice of correct catheter at the outset avoids the necessity of early change in most cases (see Urethral Catheters and Catheterization, p.27). Persistent 'blockers' do need more frequent change but these are rare.

Sending the catheter tip for laboratory culture post-removal is of no value, as the tip will have become contaminated as it is drawn through the urethra.

It is wrong to think that urine leakage from the urethra around the catheter can be stopped by passing a larger catheter and 'bunging' up the orifice with a larger balloon as it will only intensify the problem. To stop leakage, the bladder spasm caused by the catheter irritating the trigone should be treated, and a drug aimed at reducing bladder spasm (e.g. probanthine 15 mg three times a day orally) can be given, but recatheterizing with a smaller size catheter may be required to resolve the problem. Valid reasons for recatheterizing must include obstruction, contamination or malfunction.

Catheter care

Good catheter care is vital for patient comfort and to reduce infection risk. The presence of a catheter causes urethral secretion due to irritation, and this should not be allowed to dry on the catheter. Antiseptic cream, e.g. chlorhexidine 1% applied to gauze, wrapped around the catheter and firmly secured, produces an antiseptic barrier at the catheter tip, and has been shown clinically to help reduce the incidence of infection by bacteria between the catheter wall and urethra. It also prevents contamination by any in-and-out movement of the catheter.

Catheter security can be enhanced by fixing the drainage tube to the leg, usually by the use of elastoplast strapping. An antiseptic cream dressing should have a minimum daily change. This technique is slowly replacing the more traditional concept of 4-hourly catheter toilet (cleaning the tip of the penis) which results in the catheter being disturbed more frequently. Some practitioners advocate that the antiseptic cream be applied to the catheter junction and massaged into the urethra in the female patient by moving the catheter gently up and down.

While the catheter is in situ in the male patient, the foreskin must not be left retracted behind the head of the penis as this can result in painful complications, e.g. paraphimosis. The catheter must not be secured in such a way as to produce the risk of other complications, such as meatal pressure.

There is no reason to change drainage bags if they are working well. Most manufacturers give the life expectancy of a bag as about seven to ten days, although some units adopt the practice of regular 48-hourly change of urine bags in an attempt to minimize infection.

Studies have shown that wetting of the perineum, especially in female patients, can contaminate the catheter with bowel flora, so selective showers and blanket baths for catheterized patients seem to carry less risk of introducing infection.

Different jugs and gloves should be used when emptying different bags at the drainage tap. To limit cross-infection, the bags are not tipped upside down or disconnected from the catheter. The aim in emptying the bag is to prevent cross-infection and, if possible, it is best not to nurse catheterized patients in adjacent beds, but this practice is obviously difficult in a urological ward. The prevention of cross-contamination is difficult, because the drainage of the catheter limits the degree of asepsis which can be employed, and because the drainage tap opens the 'closed' system. It is logical therefore to heat disinfect measuring jugs before each use and to encourage the use of antibacterial soap in handwashing during the procedure.

Much work is in progress on the development of a disposable introducer to allow the inclusion of chlorhexidine in the urine bag following the emptying process. The inclusion of a strong antiseptic has been shown to reduce the likelihood of ascending infection.

A midstream specimen of urine should, if possible, be taken before a catheter is passed. It is a good practice to make this a standard admission procedure along with a ward test of urine.

A specimen should be taken whilst the catheter is in situ, although regular specimen taking for culture and sensitivity is generally not encouraged.

Most modern drainage bags provide a self-sealing short rubber sleeve to aid aseptic withdrawal of urine. On no account should the catheter be disconnected from the urine bag to collect a specimen, or a spigot introduced to aid collection. The occlusion of the tube for 10-15 minutes to aid specimen collection can be undertaken quite effectively by using a gate clamp below the rubber sleeve. By using an alcohol swab to wipe the rubber sleeve and aspirating urine with a syringe and needle, an uncontaminated specimen can be obtained. Wearing disposable gloves also adds a further safeguard against contamination. It is inadvisable to use a needle and syringe to puncture a plastic tubing without a rubber sleeve as it will not self-seal.

Care should be taken to label the universal container and laboratory card clearly catheter specimen of urine, not midstream specimen of urine.

The syringe and needle technique is also employed when sampling urine for 4-hourly urinalysis, as in diabetes mellitus, and most manufacturers recommend the use of blue needles for sampling.

Catheter removal

It is as easy to introduce infection at removal as at any other time so care should be taken when removing the catheter. The patient should be informed and privacy ensured. An equipment tray is required containing a disposable towel, syringe and gloves. The towel should be placed under the catheter and, following deflation of the balloon using the syringe, the catheter should be wrapped in the towel and discarded with the drainage bag. The catheter bag stand should be washed and dried before being used again.

It is not good practice to cut the side arm to allow the deflation of the balloon, as often unsterile scissors and slack technique are employed. Cutting the side arm to allow the deflation of the balloon should not be employed if the fluid cannot be withdrawn, as it is the only effective connecting point for a syringe. If the catheter cannot be removed at all, surgical removal is required, but to avoid this, various other removal methods have been suggested.

Inflating the balloon with water until it bursts has been employed, but the disadvantage of this is that small pieces of rubber may break off and create the focus for calculi formation. Injecting solutions, e.g. ether, to rot the rubber of the balloon have been suggested but this is well less used.

One of the best and most successful methods is to use the thin guide wire from a ureteric catheter or one from a long line for intravenous therapy (with the cannula removed). This is passed up the balloon channel and guided through the obstruction until the fluid escapes or the balloon bursts. This technique is performed by a skilled practitioner who has had adequate instruction and practice.

Catheters and irrigation

When no pus or blood clots are likely to interfere with the drainage of the catheter, a two-way catheter is employed. This type of catheter has two channels, one via a side arm to inflate the balloon to keep the catheter in place and one to allow urine to drain into the drainage bag.

When pus or blood clots are likely to cause a problem with drainage, a three-way catheter is used. These catheters have an extra channel to allow fluid to be run into the bladder, diluting the urine and allowing it to escape freely.

Bladder irrigation is used in theatre to enhance vision and wash away blood. Generally 3-litre sterile bags on a 'Y' type administration set are used. These are closely observed to prevent the bags emptying and air entering the system. Water is not used for irrigation because it can be absorbed by the cells, nor is normal saline because in any procedure using electricity, e.g. diathermy, electricity could be conducted through the bladder via the solution. For these reasons glycine, a non-electrolyte solution, is used.

Once the patient is back on the ward after surgery the latter problem is eliminated and a cheaper solution may be used for irrigation. Sterile normal saline, supplied in 3-litre and 1-litre bags, or less commonly sterile water is used. Irrigation fluid can be absorbed from the bladder and cause complications, a side effect which should be borne in mind.

Saline tends to be used more frequently because it is isotonic (i.e the same osmotic pressure as blood plasma) and therefore absorption of the saline could result in increased blood sodium levels. However, water absorbed from the bladder can produce the problem of haemolysis (disintegration of the red blood cells) by reducing the osmolarity of the blood. It can also be associated with cerebral oedema producing such symptoms as confusion.

It is important that a fluid chart is completed accurately with the amount of irrigation fluid entered separately from the fluid emptied from the drainage bag. The difference between the two figures is the total urine output.

Once the irrigation system is in situ it is not disturbed, to reduce the risk of infection, as with the drainage system. The irrigation fluid used is always sterile and its flow rate is governed by the depth of haematuria. It is unnecessary to run a very fast irrigation if the urine is not heavily blood-stained. The fast turbulent fluid only aggravates any 'oozy' blood vessels.

Absolute care though must be taken when governing the flow rate to avoid clot retention. General opinion now discourages the use of an 'irrigation' trolley at the foot of the bed to reduce the chance of cross-contamination.

If clots need to be removed, 'milking' rollers are sometimes employed, but milking the tube between the fingers and palms of the hand can be very effective. A bladder irrigation set with a bulb achieving a smilar effect has been suggested. This is also aimed at limiting the number of occasions disconnection is required.

Instillation

If infection is present an antiseptic solution is sometimes used to inhibit growth and reproduction of the micro-organisms. e.g. chlorhexidine (Hibitane) 0.2% (1:5000 dilution) solution as a continuous irrigation. Only rarely is it necessary to break the seal between the catheter and drainage bag deliberately. The inter-mittent instillation of antiseptic solution is not thought to be very effective in the prevention of infection. Some units do not advocate instillation at all but treat the infection by increasing fluid intake to 'flush' out any sediment or mucus, a practice which should be encouraged even if irrigation is employed.

In the presence of infection intermittent bladder instillation of antiseptic solution may be prescribed. Noxyflex (Noxythiolin) is a fairly frequently prescribed solution. One per cent solution has been shown to be as effective as 2.5% solution with a reduced incidence of associated haematuria. Generally 50 ml is instilled and held for 20 minutes before release. Chlorhexidine irrigation fluid (100 ml retained for 20 minutes twice daily) has been demonstrated to be one of the most effective/active solutions, with little effect on the lining of the urinary tract.

Although noxyflex and chlorhexidine are perhaps the most widely used irrigating solutions, the choice of irrigating fluid can be influenced by the sensitivity of the organism causing the infection, and no one solution appears to cover all the possible infecting organisms. Other solutions used in the management of urinary tract infection include:

1. Acetic acid, used as a 0.25% solution in normal saline, has a preventive effect on bacterial growth by increasing the acid environment within the bladder. However, it can cause irritation of the bladder lining even in weak solutions.

2. Amphotericin B, used mainly in the treatment of *Candida* (fungal) infections in a solution of 100 mg/l. It has never demonstrated any

clinical problems, but the drug is known to be quite toxic.

3. Povidone-iodine (Betadine), used quite extensively as an antibacterial agent. It has two major problems in its use — its high chemical activity and the danger of allergic reaction. It has not been associated with the emergence of any resistant bacterial strains, but its use has mainly been in the treatment of hospital-related (nosocomial) infections.

Although the standard practice of bladder instillation is basically the same as for bladder lavage (see p.31), many units have been looking at the technique of bladder instillation to try to improve technique. This can be achieved by using the outlet port (for sampling) as an inlet. Although this limits the life of a drainage bag, as most manufacturers recommend a use of a blue needle and a larger bore needle is required for this technique, it does minimize the number of occasions on which the catheter is disconnected. After emptying the bag and gate-clamping the tubing below the inlet port, the irrigation can be instilled using a sterile needle and syringe via the specimen port. It can be released after the allotted time without disconnecting the bag at all.

The current practice of instilling fluid by disconnecting the catheter has two problems:

1. Forceps are often employed to retain the fluid before a spigot is inserted. These can bite into the catheter material causing damage.

2. The system is 'open' on at least two occasions. It is perhaps better to re-attach the drainage bag with a gate clamp in situ to eliminate one of these occasions.

Whilst the irrigation system is in situ the patient needs to be turned to different positions to ensure overall exposure of the bladder to the solution. Patients often find antiseptic solutions difficult to tolerate as they can cause a burning sensation. It is vital to reassure and comfort the patient.

Hand irrigation

If clot retention is unavoidable, hand irrigation is required. This is an aseptic procedure requiring two people. A trolley is prepared containing:

1. Two towels.
2. Sterile receiver or jug.
3. Sterile bladder syringe.

4. Sterile gloves.

5. Irrigation solution.

6. Alcohol wipe (e.g. Steret).

7. Spigot or gate clamp for antiseptic bladder solution.

The practitioner should not handle anything unsterile once gloves are applied, and the connection should be wiped with an alcohol wipe before disconnecting. Only 30-50 ml of the fluid should be instilled and then gently drawn out through the drainage channel, to remove clots or debris. A backward and forward action on the syringe can be effective during instillation and this is continued until there is clear or clot-free fluid returned. With multiple clots a specialist often has difficulty with the procedure and re-catheterizing the patient may be required. A receiver between the legs is advisable when freeing clot retention, because as clots are freed fluid usually rushes out.

If there is any doubt about the sterility of the bag tip or there are many clots in the tubing, it is perhaps better to set up a new system. The system should be closed as quickly as possible, ensuring that there is no air lock before leaving the drainage bag, and that the fluid is draining freely.

Further reading

Blandy J P (1981) How to catheterise the bladder, British Journal of Hospital Medicine 26 (1): 58-60

Blannin J P and Hobden J (1980) The catheter of choice, Nursing Times 76 (48): 2092-2093

(1983) Catheterization and urinary tract infection, Nursing 2 (13): supplt

Harper W E S (1981) Appraisal of 12 solutions used for bladder irrigation/ instillation, British Journal of Urology 53 (5): 433-438

Jenner E A (1977) A closed system of urinary drainage, Nursing Mirror 145 (18): supplt

Jenner E A (1983) Cutting the cost of catheter infections, Nursing Times 79 (28): 58, 60-61

Kirk D et al (1979) Hibitane bladder irrigation in the prevention of catheter associated urinary infections, British Journal of Urology 51 (6): 528-531

Meers P, and Strange J L (1980) Hospital should do the sick no harm, No.7. Urinary Tract Infections, Nursing Times 76 (30): supplt

O'Conner G (1978) Catheterisation in terminally ill patients, Nursing Mirror 147 (1): supplt

(1982) Urinary tract infection, the role of the nurse, Proceedings of conference at Northwick Park Hospital (May 21, 1982)

Seal D V (1982) Southampton Infection Control Team, The inclusion of chlorhexidine in urinary drainage bags, Lancet 1 (8278): 965

Southampton Infection Control Team (1982) Evaluation of aseptic techniques and chlorhexidine on the rate of catheter-associated urinary tract infection, Lancet 1 (8263): 89-90

Strange J L (1976) Infection of the urinary tract associated with catheters, Nursing Times 72 (11): 726-727

Walsh R (1980) Urethral catheterization, British Medical Journal: 728-730

Wastling G (1978) Long term indwelling catheters, Nursing Times 74 (28): 1176-1177

Whitfield H N (1976) Non sterile intermittent self, Nursing Times 72 (50): 1961

CHAPTER 3

DISEASES OF THE PENIS

Phimosis

Phimosis is the name given to an abnormally tight prepuce (foreskin) which cannot be retracted. This condition predisposes to carcinoma of the penis.

Causes

1. Congenital.
2. Carcinoma of penis.
3. Repeated infection, causing scarring.
4. Ammonia burns.

Signs and symptoms

1. Painful erection — difficult ejaculation or painful coitus (may be The foreskin balloons out when voiding.
2. Painful erection — difficult ejaculation or painful coitus (may be dis- covered in investigation for infertility).
3. Balanitis — ulceration or oedema of prepuce due to bacterial

Treatment

Circumcision is the treatment of choice.

Paraphimosis

Paraphimosis occurs when the foreskin has been retracted behind the head of the penis but cannot be drawn forward again. The inner layer of the foreskin then forms a tight collar behind the glans preventing normal venous and lymphatic return and creating a band of oedema.

Causes

1. Following erection.
2. Retraction of the foreskin and not returning it, e.g. after instrumentation, catheterization or catheter care; mother drawing foreskin back in young child. Normal development of the foreskin takes upward of a year after birth.

Signs and symptoms

1. Inability to retract foreskin.
2. Pain.
3. Band of oedema increasing in severity as condition continues.
4. Gangrene of the glans penis may ensue if not corrected.

Treatment

1. Manipulation. Using gentle, firm pressure with a gloved hand it is sometimes possible to reduce the foreskin and dispel the oedema.
2. Injection of the oedematous collar to help dispersion before manipulation, e.g. hyaluronidase injection (Hyalase) 1500 iu subcutaneous.
3. Surgery. A dorsal slit is cut at the top of the oedematous foreskin to release the constriction and reduce the discomfort and oedema.

Preoperative preparation

1. Explain the procedure to the patient.
2. Pubic shave (if surgeon prefers).

Postoperative care

1. General observation.
2. Dressing is usually light, e.g. vaseline gauze.
3. Formal circumcision is arranged when the condition has had time to settle.

Circumcision

Circumcision is removal of the foreskin.

Reasons for operation

1. Religious belief (non-medical reason).
2. Phimosis.
3. Paraphimosis.
4. Balanitis.
5. Suspected carcinoma of penis.

Preoperative preparation

1. Explain the procedure and reassure the patient.
2. Pubic shave (if surgeon prefers).
3. Nil for local anaesthetic though general anaesthetic more usual.

Postoperative care

1. Suture care (sutures are usually catgut).
2. Dressing is usually light, e.g. paraffin gauze (tulle gras), ribbon gauze soaked in tincture benzoin (Friars Balsam).
3. Early warm salt bath; dressing allowed to float off.
4. Patient discharged first or second day if no complications occur. Often the patient complains of a forked stream. This settles without treatment.

Complications

1. Erection postoperation can be very painful. Mild sedation, anaesthetic gel and analgesia is usually sufficient for relief. Hormone therapy to reduce erection is sometimes, though rarely, used.
2. Haemorrhage.

Balanitis

Balanitis is inflammation of the surface of the head of the penis.

Causes
1. Poor hygiene.
2. Phimosis, preventing good hygiene.
3. Inadequate catheter care.
4. Urethral discharge.

Signs and symptoms
1. Discharge (often purulent).
2. Encrusted hard smegma (a sebaceous substance secreted by the glands of the glans penis).
3. Penis tip sore and irritated.
4. Red and sore glans penis.

Treatment
1. Good hygiene using soap and water or general bath with thorough cleaning of the penis.
2. Circumcision.
3. Treatment of the predisposing condition.

Complications
Recurrent balanitis predisposes to carcinoma of penis.

Peyronie's disease
Peyronie's disease is a not uncommon condition in which scar tissue is deposited in the normally spongy tissue of the penis.

Cause
Unknown

Signs and symptoms
The penis lies abnormally to one side with an obvious curve when flaccid. This does not alter during erection, making intercourse painful and uncomfortable.

Treatment
No treatment has been found to be fully effective.

Carcinoma of penis
Carcinoma of the penis is often a squamous cell type carcinoma which tends to invade the head of the penis.

Cause
The cause is unknown. There is a predisposition to carcinoma in cases of:
1. Phimosis
2. Chronic balanitis
3. Previous simple penile lesion, e.g. warts.

Signs and symptoms
1. Phimosis — tumour prevents foreskin being drawn back.
2. Small lump or ulcer felt on penis.
3. Discharge, often blood-stained.
4. Distinctive foul smell.

Treatment
1. Circumcision and biopsy.
2. Removal of penis.
3. Examination and/or lymphangiogram to assess any secondary involvement. This may necessitate lymph node dissection in the groin.
4. Radiotherapy (a) Initially if no lymphatic involvement; (b) Post-amputation as back-up treatment.

Preoperative preparation
1. The psychological well being of these patients must be considered. The stress of a disfiguring operation and its sexual effects necessitate careful counselling and explanation.
2. Pubic shave.
3. No other special physical preparation.

Postoperative care The aim is to maintain the patient's comfort. Dressings tend to ooze and need regular attention. A catheter is often left in situ for 7 - 10 days. After catheter removal the patient will generally void sitting down.

Lymph node dissection, if required, makes nursing care more difficult because lymph tends to leak under the wound which often becomes red and hard, and frequently the suture line parts at some point.

The groin is full of creases, and difficult to dress due to constant movement. Padding becomes wet, which is ineffective and uncomfortable. The skin must be protected from irritant discharge — 'skin prep' protective application is very effective for this purpose. The fluid must be collected — flange-less drainage bags, e.g. Coloplast, are often very useful.

Penile warts

Penile warts may be small, single growths but, if untreated, can increase in number. It is more usual for warts to appear in crops. The treatment of this condition often falls within the scope of the venereologist.

Causes

Penile warts are usually venereal in origin, commonly caused by viral infection, e.g. Verruca vulgaris.

Treatment

Penile warts are removed by

1. Fulguration (diathermy).
2. Surgery.
3. Liquid nitrogen.
4. Application of podopyllum resin (Podophyllin). This compound is painted onto the warts, left up to 6 hours and then washed off. It is quite a toxic solution, and must be used in small amounts, taking care to avoid the surrounding tissues.

Preoperative preparation

No special preparation

Postoperative care

General observation

Priapism

Priapism is a prolonged, painful erection which is not associated with any sexual influence. Males of any age can be affected.

Causes

Diseases which can predispose to priapism include:

1. Blood disorders, e.g. sickle cell disease.
2. Neurological diseases, e.g. spinal cord injury, cerebrovascular accident.

Treatment

Priapism requires urological treatment within about 30 hours of onset to prevent complications. Treatment includes:

1. Analgesia, e.g. morphine.
2. Cold compress as a first aid measure.
3. Surgical intervention to relieve venous congestion.

Complications

1. Fibrosis of erectile tissue.
2. Impotence.
3. Impairment of future erection.

Further reading

(1983) Clinical insight, hypospadias, Nursing Mirror 156 (2):supplt

Oriel J D (1983) Genital warts, British Journal of Sexual Medicine 10 (96): 44-45

Pryor J P (1982) Priapism, Practitioner 226 (1373): 1873-1879

CHAPTER 4

URETHRAL CONDITIONS

Hypospadias

Hypospadias is a malformation in which the urethra opens onto the underside of the penis. It is congenitally determined. Hypospadias may cause infection, infertility (sperm cannot be delivered to the correct place) or obstructions if the opening becomes narrowed.

Treatment

Surgery (often the Denis Browne operation) is usually performed early in life. Stage 1 (at 2-3 years old) straightens the penis, and Stage 2 (at 5-7 years old) reconstructs the urethra.

Epispadias

Epispadias is a malformation in which the urethra opens onto the upper side of the penis.

Treatment

Treatment is the same as for hypospadias.

Urethritis

Urethritis is inflammation of the urethral lining. It is often acute but it may become chronic in nature, with acute episodes. It is often associated with urine infection usually in female patients.

Causes

1. Catheterization/instrumentation.

2.   Chemical irritant, e.g. from catheter lining.
3.   Phimosis.
4.   Pre-existing urinary tract infection.
5.   Sexually transmitted. A non-gonococcal venereal disease usually viral in origin — non specific urethritis. Symptoms of gonorrhoea begin with profound urethritis. The patient is usually referred to a venereologist.

Signs and symptoms

1.   Pain and burning sensation on micturition, 'broken glass sensation'.
2.   Tenderness and irritation.
3.   Dysuria.
4.   Frequency.
5.   Urethral discharge.
6.   Haematuria.
7.   Casts in the urine.
8.   Vaginal irritation, if chronic in nature.
9.   Pyrexia and signs of generalized infection, if severe.

Investigations

1.   Midstream specimen of urine.
2.   Routine ward test of urine.

Treatment

1.   Encourage the patient to take oral fluids.
2.   Broad-spectrum antibiotic.

Complications
Urethral stricture.

Urethral stricture
Urethral stricture is a narrowing of the urethra, it can affect any part and be of any length. It more commonly affects the bulbous part of the urethra (near its point of entry into the bladder).

Causes

1. Urethritis.
2. Indwelling catheter.
3. Trauma, e.g. fracture of pelvis, foreign body.
4. Catheterization.
5. Instrumentation/cystoscopy.
6. Surgical complications, e.g. prostatectomy, hypospadias repair.
7. Obstetric complication, e.g. following childbirth.
8. Congenital (rare).
9. Venereal disease.
10. Tumour (rare).

Signs and symptoms

Lower tract obstruction:

1. Difficulty in starting stream.
2. Thin stream, but often forceful (unlike prostatic obstruction).
3. Forked stream.
4. Postmicturition dribbling, dribbling incontinence.
5. Chronic retention.
6. Feeling of incomplete bladder emptying.
7. Infection — Dysuria } All other symptoms related to urinary
    Frequency } tract infection.
8. Retention of urine, acute or chronic. In either case a suprapubic catheter is sometimes passed initially to avoid possible catheterization difficulties.

Investigations

1. Midstream specimen of urine.
2. Cysto-urethroscopy.
3. Micturating cystogram.
4. Intravenous urogram.
5. Urethrogram.

6. Cystometry.
7. Blood test for venereal disease.

Treatment
1. Dilatation of the urethra.
2. Internal urethrotomy.
3. Urethroplasty.
4. Meatoplasty.

The patient is usually advised to avoid exercises involving a straddle position, e.g. cycling.

Constipation is avoided to prevent unnecessary irritation of stricture. Other problems involve retention of urine.

Dilatation of the urethra

Dilators gradually increasing in diameter are passed down the urethra to open out the stricutre. This procedure is often performed as a day case, and may be performed under local anaesthetic although general anaesthetic is more usual. Epidural anaesthesia is sometimes employed. Metal dilators, 'bougies', are most often used although dilators vary in construction and design — many surgeons have their own preference (Fig. 9).

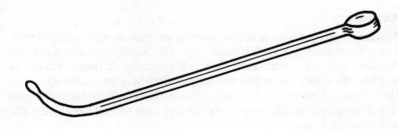

Figure   9. Diagram of urethral dilator (bougie)

No specific preparation is required, except that for the type of anaesthesia to be used.

Gradually, larger and larger dilators are gently manipulated through the stricture until the urethra is opened out to allow good urine stream. They are not forced because of the danger of trauma. Lubrication is normally employed using an anaesthetic/mucosal disinfectant preparation, e.g. instillagel, or lignocaine gel.

Postoperatively, the following measure are taken:

1. General observation.
2. Ensure micturition, especially in patients admitted as day cases.
3. Encourage the patient to take oral fluids.
4. Repeat 'bouginage' is almost always required, initially fortnightly or monthly, decreasing to 6-monthly intervals.

Complications of dilatation

1. Haemorrhage.
2. Further fibrosis of urethra.
3. Restricture.
4. False passage formation.
5. Ruptured urethra (fistula).
6. Infection. Severe development include bacteraemia and septicaemia. bacteraemia and septicaemia.

Urethrotomy

Urethrotomy is an operation to slit the urethral stricture along its upper length. The instrument used is a urethrotome (Fig. 10), which is passed down the urethra to the stricture, a retractable blade is advanced to cut the stricture and a lens machanism allows the surgeon to see exactly where he is cutting.

This method of treatment of strictures is sometimes preferred as it eliminates the 'blind' technique of dilatation and strictures seem to heal better than after forcing a stricture open.

Reasons for urethrotomy

1. Surgeon's preference.

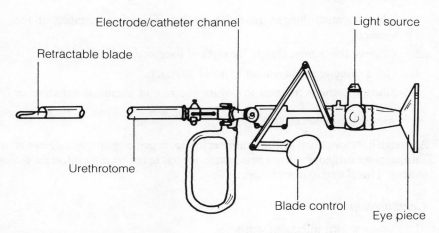

Figure 10. Diagram of a urethrotome with a retractable blade

2. Narrow strictures in patients requiring cystoscopy/resection, to enable passage of the instrument.
3. Strictures not responding to dilatation.
4. Strictures unsuitable for urethroplasty.

The main contra-indication to urethrotomy is urinary tract infection, as performing the technique under infective conditions can cause sepsis or severe haemorrhage.

Preoperative care

1. Mid-stream specimen of urine — elimination of urinary tract infection is vital.
2. Antibiotic therapy, if infection is present.
3. Pubic shave, if surgeon prefers.
4. Routine preparation for general anaesthetic.

Postoperative care

1. Routine observations
2. Urinary catheter is situ (usually for about 7 days although some surgeons

advocate much longer, from 3-6 weeks). This allows healing of the incision.

3. Observe the patient closely for signs of haemorrhage and blockage.

4. Good catheter management to avoid infection.

5. Silicone catheter is used to reduce the risk of chemical irritation or urethritis.

6. Antibiotics (if necessary).

Although it is more usual to find a catheter in situ, depending upon the degree of cutting, some surgeons will not pass a catheter so as to reduce discomfort for the patient. This is uncommon, however.

Complications

1. Urinary tract infection, sepsis.

2. Haemorrhage.

Urethroplasty

Urethroplasty, usually a two stage operation, is designed to restore a strictured urethra to a patent tube. It is a difficult operation to describe simply.

Stage one

Preoperative preparation Preoperative care is the same as for urethrotomy. Cleansing of the perineal area with antiseptic soap is essential.

Procedure The strictured urethra is exposed and then excised, leaving the epithelial tissue at the bed of the urethra exposed. This epithelial tissue is then sutured to the cut edges of the skin (epithelium). A perineal opening is left to allow the patient to void sitting down. The raw tissue is left for at least 12 weeks to allow the two epithelial surfaces to knit together well and to be secure enough to withstand further surgery.

Postoperative care

1. Routine observations.

2. Urine catheter sometimes in situ (occasionally suprapubic).

3. Careful observation and care of dressing; infection of the wound is an obvious hazard due to the general area and nature of surgery.

Stage two

Preoperative preparation

1. Mid-stream specimen of urine check
2. Careful preoperative cleansing.

Procedure Going beyond the line of healing a wider oval area of tissue is cut, rolled into a tube and sutured over a catheter. The skin edges that remain are drawn together and sutured over the new tube that has been fashioned. A dorsal slit may be required to relax the skin tension.

Postoperative care

1. The patient is catheterized for 7-10 days (to allow the scar to heal).
2. Catheter specimens of urine are taken regularly for culture.
3. There is careful monitoring and care of dressing.

Urethral trauma

Urethral trauma occurs more frequently in men than women.

Causes

1. Passing stones.
2. Instrumentation.
3. External injury, e.g. falling straddle over an object, pelvic girdle injury damaging the urethra.
4. Multiple injury.
5. Rupture caused by pressure due to stricture (very rare).
6. In women, long labour, pressure on urethra, damage with delivery forceps.

Signs and symptoms

1. Bleeding via the urethra.
2. Inability to pass urine.
3. Shock.
4. Signs of leak into scrotum, abdominal wall or perineum.

Diagnosis

1. Rectal examination.
2. Urethral Bleeding.
3. Urethrogram.
4. Inability to pass urine.

Treatment

Suprapubic catheterization is sometimes performed to allow repair naturally.

Most urologists advocate performing a urethrogram before the insertion of a urethral catheter if they suspect urethral rupture. Sometimes if urethral catheterization is preferable, it is performed under direct vision with the use of a urethroscope in the operating theatre. The patient may also require relief of collection outside the urinary tract.

Surgical repair

Urethroplasty. Urethral tears generally heal with some degree of stricture and surgical intervention is often required.

Meatotomy (meatoplasty)

Meatotomy is a simple operation used to relieve a stricture at the opening of the penis. The opening is made larger using scissors and the cut ends sutured to enhance the wider opening.

Preoperative care

Pubic shave (if surgeon prefers)

Postoperative care

1. Sutures are usually made of dissolvable catgut.
2. Salt bath, daily for at least 5 days, aids healing and maintains hygiene.
3. The operated penile opening is inspected daily and gently probed to prevent the raw edges from sticking together. The patient is taught to do this himself after initiating the treatment. (The nozzle from the end of the lignocaine gel tube is often used to good effect.) The patient may complain that the urine stream is not straight but this subsides as the operation settles.

Further reading

Blandy J (1978) Urethral stricture in the male, Nursing Mirror 147 (6): 13-16

Desmond A D (1981) Evaluation of direct vision urethrotomy, British Journal of Urology 53 (6): 630-632

Scott E (1977) One stage urethroplasty (Nursing Care Study), Nursing Mirror 145 (9): 16-18

Smith P J B (1983a) Urethral syndrome 1, British Journal of Sexual Medicine 10 (95): 30-34

Smith P J B (1983b) Urethral syndrome 2, British Journal of Sexual Medicine 10 (96):13-18

CHAPTER 5

TESTICULAR SURGERY AND
SCROTAL CONDITIONS

The testes normally develop in the abdomen and then descend into the scrotum via the inguinal canal during foetal development at about the thirty-sixth week. They are therefore in place at birth. This is why a midwife feels for both testes in the scrotum during the examination of the baby soon after birth. Occasionally the testes do take a little longer to descend into the scrotum after birth, so the examination of children at school includes examination of testes.

Retractile testis

A retractile testis has not descended properly from the inguinal canal into the scrotum. Manipulation sometimes allows the testes to be moved into the correct position. If this works, no surgery is performed, but if the testis is high in the scrotum and cannot be moved, surgery is necessary to prevent the possible complications.

Ectopic testis

If the testis deviates from the normal line of descent, it will finish in a place other than the scrotum. This can happen because of a barrier of tissue. Surgery early in the child's development is needed to replace the testis in the scrotum, otherwise complications may arise. Positions in which the testis can occur are penile, perineal or femoral, but most commonly in the superficial inguinal pouch.

Undescended testis

Often associated with a hernia, the condition is treated early in a child's life, and the hernia is repaired at the same time. The testis does not develop normally when undescended.

Undescended testes can affect fertility because the tubules within the testes producing the sperm do not mature properly. The condition can be painful and can slightly increase the chance of malignant change.

Treatment

The operation to replace the testis in its correct position in the scrotum is called orchidopexy. The operation is usually done at an early age, often before 6 years of age so that the spermatic cord can grow with the child.

Postoperative care   No special postoperative care is generally required. Holding the testis in place is normally achieved by internal fixation at surgery. The testis may be missing or if it is abnormal, it is removed. A Silastic implant resembling the normal anatomy is sometimes inserted for psychological reasons. Prognosis with early surgery is good.

Torsion of testis

Torsion of the testis is a surgical emergency. The testis is suspended by mesentery (mesorchium) which can twist if there is a congenital abnormality allowing excessive mobility of the testis. Torsion can occur in newborn babies. The twisting is the torsion (volvulus) and it will interfere with the blood supply to the testis causing initial discomfort and leading to gangrene requiring orchidectomy if not treated quickly. This condition is most commonly seen in young men aged 13 - 16 years. The patient may have had warning signs in the form of periods of discomfort which resolve spontaneously. The condition can mimic other conditions such as epididymo-orchitits or strangulated inguinal hernia.

Causes

1.   Congenital abnormality.
2.   Undescended testes.
3.   Trauma.

Signs and symptoms

1. Acute pain — referred to groin and lower abdomen (can mimic renal colic closely).
2. Tenderness.
3. Swelling.
4. Redness.
5. Nausea, sometimes vomiting.

Treatment

Emergency surgery in theatre to correct the vascular obstructions and securing the testicle to reduce mobility and prevent re-occurrence. The unaffected testicle must be fixed in the scrotum at the same time as it is very prone to torsion at a later date.

Preoperative preparation

1. Pubic shave.
2. Analgesia.
3. No special preparation is required.

Postoperative care

1. Analgesia.
2. Scrotal support.

Complications

Gangrene of testis.

Testicular tumour

Testicular tumour is a rare condition which arises in two main forms.

1. Seminoma, usually appears in patients aged 30-40 years. It is fairly slow growing and secondary deposits take quite a time to develop.
2. Teratoma, usually appears in patients aged 20-30 years. It tends to have rapid growth with early development of secondary deposits.

These tumours spread initially via the lymphatic system to the nodes in the lumbar region and can eventualy produce secondary deposits in many areas, most commonly the liver and lung. Local spread is rare unless the scrotum is punctured.

Cause

The cause is unknown, but it may be predisposed by undescended testes.

Signs and symptoms

1. The size of the testicle increases. This is the factor bringing most cases to medical attention.
2. Discomfort in groin due to increased weight.
3. Hardness.
4. Pain, e.g. if bleeding.
5. Redness/oedema of scrotum with secondary deposits. It can present like acute epididymo-orchitis but does not resolve.
6. Persistent backache — secondary deposits via lymphatic system.
7. Gynaecomastia (breast development) ⎫
    Dyspnoea   ⎬ Secondary deposits
    Dry cough   ⎬ in lung
    Haemoptysis   ⎭

Investigations

Clinical history and examination   Diagnosis is obtained by high inguinal orchidectomy (not biopsy-local spread) and examination of remaining testicle.

For spread

1. Chest x-ray.
2. Examination of abdomen for palpable lymph nodes, e.g. pelvis, liver.
3. Examination for gynaecomastia/nipple tenderness.

Investigations or teratoma

Because of the extent of treatment for teratoma, extensive investigations are required:

1. Histology review

2. Whole lung tomography

3. Lymphangiogram

4. Intravenous pyelogram, e.g. for displaced ureters

5. Liver scan

6. Liver and abdominal ultrasound

7. Haemoglobin, full blood count, urea and electrolytes

8. Tomogram of abdomen and thorax

9. Computerized whole body tomogram

10. Human chorionic gonadotrophin and alphafectoprotein. These are produced by these tumours and are used as a guide to treatment response.

11. Kidney function tests — cytotoxic drugs are very nephrotoxic so good kidney function is essential.

12. Lung function test

Treatment

Seminoma Once the tumour is removed, a lymphangiogram is usually performed to establish whether there is any spread. Seminomas are usually very sensitive to radiotherapy. Treatment with 4 - 6 weeks radiotherapy is usually performed postorchidectomy.

Teratoma Teratoma are very much more difficult to treat. They are less radio-sensitive and recent treatment usually combines both radiotherapy and chemotherapy. The treatment using chemotherapy is normally initiated in a specialized unit experienced in this work. Because of the age of the patient involved, a medical social worker help is almost always sought to help with family and financial responsibilities

Stage 1   testis only — radiotherapy for about 3 weeks

Stage 2(a)   testis with lymph nodes under 2 cm diameter — radiotherapy for about $3\frac{1}{2}$ weeks and a further course after one month's rest

		Four courses of chemotherapy (Einhorn
Stage 2(b)	testis with lymph nodes 2 - 5 cm diameter	therapy), then radiotherapy.
Stage 2(c)	testis with lymph nodes above 5 cm diameter	Surgery is
Stage 3	lymph nodes involved above diaphrahm	sometimes performed.
Stage 4	multiple secondary deposits	Maximum of six courses of chemotherapy

Sperm banking may be employed in the hope of providing children once treatment is complete.

Einhorn therapy Einhorn therapy is a 16-day chemotherapeutic course repeated every 3 weeks. The first 5 days of the course are given in hospital, the remainder is given as outpatient (if the patient is well enough). Hydration of the patient is necessary before drugs are started because of the toxicity of platinum.

Investigations undertaken include:

1. Alphafetoprotein determination.

2. Human chorionic gonadotrophin determination

3. Ethylene diamine tetra-acetate clearance test (ethylene-diamine tetra-acetic acid is used to determine whether renal function is good before treatment is started because platinum is highly nephrotoxic)

4. Liver function tests.

5. Height and weight measurements because drug doses are calculated according to the patient's surface area.

The hydration procedure consists of 1 litre normal saline and 2g potassium chloride given intravenously for at least 12 hours before chemotherapy begins and continued for 5 days.

The therapeutic procedure consists of:

1. Cis platinum: $20\,mg/m^2$ intravenously in 100 ml of normal saline over 15 minutes on days 1,2,3,4 and 5 of course.

2. Vinblastine: 0.2 mg/kg intravenously as bolus on days 1 and 2 of course only.

3. Bleomycin: 30 mg intravenously as bolus injection on days 2, 9 and 16 of course.

4. Blood tests: Haemoglobin, full blood count, alphaetoprotein and human chorionic gonadotrophin levels measured twice weekly during treatment.

5. 4-hourly temperature, pulse and respiration: There is a danger of leuco-penia (decreased number of white blood cells) with cytotoxic drugs.

6. Analgesia: for muscle pain (myalgia).

7. Frequent mouth care: patients are susceptible to mouth infection

8. Fluid balance chart: accurate urine monitoring due to cis platinum effects.

9. Anti-emetics: Cis platinum administration is often associated with nausea and vomiting.

Orchidectomy

Orchidectomy is the removal of a testicle or testicles.

Reasons for operation

1. Tumour, e.g. testicular, prostate (to diminish hormonal activity)

2. Gangrene, e.g. as a result of torsion

3. Undescended testicle, e.g. if orchidopexy impossible

4. Atrophy

5. Severe abscess

6. Infected hydrocele

7. Tuberculosis

8. Hernia (inguinal) repair

Preoperative preparation

There is no special preparation. Shaving is required, usually for inguinal inci-sion. A scrotal incision is normally employed for orchidectomy in the treatment of prostatic cancer (subcapsular orchidectomy) Reassure the patient that fertil-ity is not reduced by loss of a testicle.

Postoperative care

1. No special postoperative care is required
2. Drain sometimes needed for 24-48 hours
3. Scrotal support
4. Scrotal sutures to skin if inserted are usually catgut to avoid the difficult removal of non-dissolving closures.

Complications

Damage to remaining testicular vessels and vas deferens infection.

Varicocele

Varicocele is varicosity of the veins of the testicle. It occurs more often on the left side than on the right.

Causes

1. Usually unknown
2. Secondary to tumour
3. Secondary to left renal carcinoma blocking left renal vein where left testicular vein enters

Signs and symtoms

1. Scrotal swelling which disappears when the patient is lying down
2. Ache or discomfort (rare)
3. Most often discovered during routine physical examination, or in the investigation of infertility problems.
4. Infertility. The blood in the veins causes a heat increase reducing sperm motility.

Treatment

1. Conservative — supportive bandage.
2. Operative — surgical ligation — varicocelectomy by tying the main feeding vein close to the inguinal canal, usually under general anaesthetic.

Preoperative preparation Groin shave.

Postoperative care Scrotal support.

Hydrocele

Hydrocele is an increased secretion and collection of serous fluid between the layers covering the testicle (tunica vaginalis).

Causes

1. In the majority of cases the cause is unknown
2. Congenital
3. Trauma
4. Neoplasm
5. Inflammation — orchitis, epididymo-orchitis.

Signs and symptoms

Hydrocele is asymptomatic in most cases. It is usually only its size and the discomfort the patient suffers that makes the patient seek help. The doctor usually confirms diagnosis by shining a light against the scrotum (transillumination).

Treatment

1. Aspiration of the fluid using a trocar and cannula.
2. Surgery — the sac in which the fluid collects is eliminated by surgery to prevent re-occurrence.

Preoperative preparation No special preparation is required

Postoperative care Patient often has a corrugated drain in situ. Scrotal support is vital.

Complications

1. Re-occurrence (if aspiration only performed)
2. Haematoma
3. Oedema of scrotum
4. Retention of urine

Haematocele

Haematocele is a collection of blood between the layers of the testicle. It is not very common.

Causes

1. Trauma
2. Tumour
3. Complication of hydrocele or other scrotal surgery
4. Torsion of testis

Signs and symptoms

1. Enlargement of scrotum
2. Bruising
3. Pain

Treatment

Examination and evacuation under general anaesthetic

Preoperative preparation Pubic shave

Postoperative care

1. Analgesia
2. Drain may be left in situ
3. Scrotal support

Complications

1. Orchidectomy may be required
2. Testicular atrophy
3. Sepsis

N.B. It is often after injury that a patient presents with a history of a scrotal swelling which he relates to the injury, but turns out to be a tumour.

Scrotal supports

As will have been noted scrotal supports are employed in nearly all cases of scrotal/testicular disease, from mild inflammation to most types of surgery. They provide much comfort and can prevent scrotal haematoma.

Orchitis

Orchitis is inflammation of the testis, usually caused by spread of a disease already present, e.g.

1. Secondary to existing infection, e.g. mumps, venereal disease carried in the blood stream to the testicle.

2. Extension of epidiymitis to epididymo-orchitis, due to urinary tract infection, tuberculosis, urethritis, infection in genito-urinary tract.

It may occur due to trauma or lesion but this is rare. It can occur at any age.

Signs and symptoms

1. Scrotal pain and tenderness which can lead to back and lower abdominal pain

2. Swollen and tender scrotum

3. High temperature; if severe, rigor

4. Scrotal oedema

5. In severe cases, nausea and vomiting

Treatment

1. Bed rest

2. Scrotal support:
    a. Scrotum supported on a cotton wool pad held in place with 3 inch Elastoplast strapping over thighs
    b. Scrotal supporter when mobile (2 -3 weeks)

3. Observe for any abscess formation

4. Analgesia

5. Antibiotic treatment with broad spectrum antibiotic (this is commenced even though the causative organism may not be known)

6. Mid-stream specimen of urine

7. 4-hourly temperature, pulse and respiration

Complications

Complications are rare. This condition usually resolves in a few days. Fibrosis can occur which will cause the sperm tubules to fail. If both sides are affected, sterility will result. Atrophy of the testes, usually when mumps caused the orchitis, can rarely happen. Hydrocele may occur.

Epididymitis

Epididymitis is inflammation of the epididymis due to infection, which can either be blood borne or occur as an extension of other genito-urinary tract infection. It occurs mainly in the older age group. It can and often does spread to the testis, producing epididymo-orchitis. It can be acute, or chronic often with acute episodes.

Causes

1. Extension of infection of urinary tract, e.g. cystitis
2. Instrumentation of genito-urinary tract, e.g. cystoscopy
3. Post-prostatectomy
4. Prolonged catheter drainage
5. Venereal disease — usually gonorrhoea (rare)
6. Tuberculosis

Signs and symptoms

1. Sudden pain — often referred to groin and lower abdomen
2. Swelling
3. Tenderness
4. Pyrexia (more rarely rigor)
5. Headache and general malaise
6. Urethral discharge sometimes
7. Hydrocele sometimes

Investigations

1. Midstream specimen of urine
2. Full urological investigation in chronic condition to isolate underlying cause, e.g. intravenous/pyelogram/urogram

3. Ensure, if a young patient, it is not testicular torsion or neoplasm
4. Chest x-ray, to exclude tuberculosis
5. Blood culture, if infection is suspected of being blood borne

Treatment

1. Bed rest
2. Scrotal support (as for orchitis)
3. Antibiotic therapy
4. Analgesia
5. Encourage the patient to take oral fluids
6. Scrotal supporter when mobilizing, usually 2 - 3 weeks
7. Reassure the patient
8. 4-hourly temperature, pulse and respiration

Complications

1. Testicular atrophy
2. Subfertility

Epididymal cyst

Epididymal cyst is a cavity which becomes filled with fluid usually near th
upper part of the epididymis. The fluid it contains can be clear or milky if sperm
enter (spermatocele). Cysts may be multiple and/or bilateral, and occur mainl
in adults.

Cause
Unknown

Signs and symptoms

1. Firm, but painless, scrotal swelling
2. Large testes
3. Dragging sensation due to testis weight
4. Awkward dressing
5. Chaffing of inner thigh skin

6.   Pain

Treatment

1.   None, unless symptoms present
2.   Excision

Preoperative preparation

1.   Routine preparation for general anaesthetic
2.   Pubic shave

Postoperative care No special postoperative care except scrotal support.

Complications

1.   Sterility
2.   Infection
3.   Haematocele

Groin or scrotal rash

Rashes in the groin or scrotal area are not uncommon. They tend to appear in the many folds of skin in this region. They generally occur in the more incapacitated, fat, or sweaty patients. Diabetics are also prone to this type of infection.

The causative organism is often a fungal infection, *Candida albicans* or thrush, and this should be confirmed by laboratory culture.

Treatment

1.   Use of the appropriate paint or dry powder spray, e.g. povidone iodine
2.   Keep the area washed, clean and well dried
3.   Prevent cross-contamination

Cream preparations tend to trap moisture in the skin which delays recovery and they are therefore not often used in the treatment of these rashes.

Sebaceous cysts of scrotum

Sebaceous cysts of scrotum are fairly common, usually small in size and rarely cause trouble

Treatment

Enucleation under local anaesthetic to avoid complications.

Complications

1. Infection
2. Calcification
3. Ulceration

Vasectomy

Vasectomy is the division of the vas deferens on both sides, performed under local or general anaesthetic.

Reasons for operation

1. Voluntary sterilization
2. Prevention of congenital illness
3. Post-prostatectomy to prevent infection

Preoperative preparation

Consent of both partners is required. Reversal is difficult so that it is vital the operation is fully understood. It is important that the marriage has a sound basis and that it is entered into with foresight. It is unusual for the operation to be performed on males under 30 years, and is often performed as a day case.

Postoperative care

1. Scrotal support and rest
2. Dissolving sutures are usually used for skin
3. Analgesia — painful testis postoperation is usual for a few days
4. Advise recommencing sexual relations fairly quickly following surgery
5. Recommend alternative contraceptive methods until semen is sperm-free
6. Regular postoperative semen analysis to check for sperm reduction in semen

Complications

1. Bruising
2. Infection
3. Sperm granuloma — if sperm leak out of the tied end of the vas, they can form a painful swelling requiring excision
4. Recanalization of vas deferens — pregnancy is usually first indication that this has occurred

Reversal of vasectomy

Reversal of vasectomy is the restoration of the spermatic channels.

Reasons for operation

1. Remarriage
2. To replace child deceased since operation
3. Changed circumstances, e.g. financial

Preoperative preparation

1. Pubic shave
2. Stress to the patient the chances of success (about 30%), provided there is good facility for anastamosis fairly recently post-vasectomy, but this declines with increase in years post-vasectomy

Postoperative care

1. 24-48 hour bed rest
2. Scrotal support
3. A suture (a nylon splint) may be left in situ, emerging throught the scrotum, its removal is required about 10 days postoperation
4. Semen analysis for viable sperm count. Samples are usually collected for examination from about two months postoperation. Auto immunity to sperm can sometimes cause infertility even after successful reversal of vasectomy.

Further reading

Allan W R (1982) The testis; torsion and trauma, Practitioner 226 (1373): 1837-1844

Ansell W (1980) A combined therapeutic approach (treatment of testicular tumours), Nursing Mirror 151 (20): 22-24

Falconer W (1979) Testicular teratoma (Nursing Care Study), Nursing Mirror 148 (19): 41-44

Jenkins I L Blacklock N J (1979) Experience with vasovasostomy; operative technique and results, British Journal of Urology 51 (1): 43-45

Johnston J H (1979) The acute scrotum in childhood, Practitioner 223 (1335): 306-310

Kelly J (1981) Teratoma (Nursing Care Study), Nursing Mirror 152 (20): 33-34

Oliver R T D (1982) Progress in the management of testicular germ-cell tumours, Practitioner 226 (1373): 1903-1915

Sewell I A (1981a) Examination of the scrotum and its contents — 1, Hospital Update 7 (2): 149-158

Sewell I A (1981b) Examination of the scrotum and its contents — 2, Hospital Update 7 (3): 297-304

Tutton E (1982) Testicular hydrocele (Nursing Care Study), Nursing Mirror 154 (13): 49

Wales H (1980) Haematoma of the scrotum (Nursing Care Study), Nursing Mirror 151 (22): 44-46

Whitaker R H (1982a) Torsion of the testes, British Journal of Hospital Medicine 27 (1): 66-69

Whitaker R H (1982b) Benign testicular swellings, Practitioner 226 (1373): 1851—1859

CHAPTER 6

PROSTATIC DISEASES

Prostatic diseases form a very important area of urology. Surgery and other treatment of prostatic disease take up much of the care in this area.
There are three main conditions treated:

1. Prostatitis
2. Benign prostatic hypertrophy
3. Carcinoma of prostate.

Prostatitis

Prostatitis is inflammation of the prostate gland, due to bacterial infection; it may be acute and/or chronic in nature.

Causes

1. Sexually transmitted disease
2. Tuberculosis
3. Local spread from disease already present, e.g. urinary tract infection cystitis, urethritis
4. Allergic reaction, e.g. asthma
5. Previous instrumentation or catheterization contamination
6. Predisposition by e.g. diabetes

Signs and symptoms

1. Frequency of voiding

2. Dysuria
3. Haematuria
4. Pyrexia, rigor
5. Burning on micturition
6. 'Smelly' urine
7. Sometimes retention of urine

Investigations

1. Per rectum examination
2. Midstream specimen of urine
3. Ward test of urine (protein)

Treatment

1. Bed rest
2. Hourly oral fluids
3. Antibiotic therapy, usually initially intramuscularly, then orally
4. Catheterization in event of retention of urine
5. With a deep seated infection, antibiotics may be ineffective and resection of tissue may be performed

Complications

1. Abscess formation
2. Urethral stricture
3. Epididymitis
4. Prostatic calculi

Benign prostatic hypertrophy

Benign prostatic hypertrophy is the most common urological condition in the adult male, affecting 35% of men over 45 years, mostly in Europe and North America. Most patients present with no symptoms. This condition is sometimes called benign prostatic hyperplasia.

Cause

The cause is unknown, but is thought to be either:

1. Advancing age causing stimulation of the disease process due to disturbance in testicular sex hormone production
2. Benign neoplasm of the gland, a fibromyo-adenoma, producing bladder outlet obstruction known as prostatism.

Signs and symptoms

Signs and symptoms include in varying degrees:

1. Start of micturition difficult and strained
2. Hesitancy (as opposed to difficult, strained commencement)
3. Poor stream
4. Frequency, especially at night (nocturia)
5. Dysuria
6. Urgency
7. Terminal dribbling
8. Incontinence (involuntary leak of urine due to abnormal bladder utlet shape)
9. Haematuria (rare)
10. Retention of urine

Acute retention of urine

Acute urine retention produces severe pain and an urgent desire to void.

Causes (other than benign prostatic hypertrophy)

1. Prostatic enlargement — cancer
2. Urethral stricture
3. Postoperative retention
4. Uterine disease in female patients
5. Neurogenic disease — injury/disease of spinal cord or sensory nerves, e.g. disseminated sclerosis
6. Hysteria

7.   Meatal ulcer with scabbing
8.   Spinal anaesthesia
9.   Blood clot retention
10. Rupture of the urethra
11. Faecal impaction
12. Acute urethritis/prostatitis
13. Urethral calculi
14. Phimosis (paraphimosis)
15. Drugs, e.g. sedatives or drugs affecting the autonomic nervous system e.g. probantheline bromide (Probanthine)
16. Muscular atony
17. Bladder calculi

Treatment of retention of urine

1.   Pain relief
2.   Catheterize the patient and prepare for surgery
3.   If there is difficulty in catheterizing the patient, it may be necessary to use a strong catheter, e.g. Simplastic, with a special tip, e.g. Coude. This may be introduced using a catheter introducer, e.g. Merryfield. A suprapubic catheter may be necessary
4.   If the patient is fit for general anaesthesia, surgery is performed. If the patient is not suitable for general anaesthesia, it may be possible to operate under epidural anaesthesia
5.   If surgery is impossible, then an indwelling catheter is used. The follow-up in the community and good catheter care are very important

Suprapubic catheterization is sometimes the treatment of choice at the outset to prevent any complications which could arise from poor urethral catheterization or trauma to the enlarged prostate.

These patients are often difficult to catheterize, so it is important that catheterization is performed by a skilled practitioner to avoid complications of urethral catheterization, which inlcude:

1.   Urinary tract infection which can seriously affect surgery
2.   Urethral stricture

3. Creation of false urethral passage
4. Severe haemorrhage
5. Ruptured urethra
6. Urethritis/cystitis.

Chronic retention of urine

Chronic retention of urine occurs when there has been long standing residual urine in the bladder even after voiding. It can produce complications:

1. Bladder — strain on bladder muscle (trabeculation)
   — diverticulum
   — acute/chronic cystitis due to stasis of urine
   — calculi formation
2. Ureter — hydroureter
3. Kidney — hydronephrosis
   — pyelonephrosis
   — pyelonephritis
   — renal failure
   — uraemia

On insertion of the catheter and in the initial phase it is important that the catheter is released very slowly to prevent any complications such as reactionary haemorrhage, shock, or renal failure due to sudden bladder decompression. These patients may also have their condition complicated by uraemia (high blood urea) due to poor excretion. It may be necessary to correct their electrolyte balance early after admission and take advice from medical/anaesthetic staff before surgery is undertaken.

Patients with symptoms who visit their general practitioner are usually referred to a urologist who will examine the patient, take a detailed history and perform a rectal examination (the prostate gland can be felt, usually smooth and round, to determine a prostatic disorder.

Surgical treatment is usually indicated if there is:

1. Residual urine
2. Upper urological tract involvement
3. Bladder disease

4.   Persistent urinary symptoms

Many patients are old and alone, they may be frightened of doctors/hospitals and afflicted with other diseases. These factors can lead to the patient delaying or avoiding medical attention early in the disease process.

Admission to urology ward

It is important that the patient:

1.   Is put in main ward and does not feel isolated. Isolation (i.e. side ward) will only serve to increase fear, anxiety and uncertainty.

2.   Is allowed visitors at any time to allay any anxiety

3.   Is allowed to have "a pint" if he enjoys one. It often helps break down any barrier.

The psychological well being of the patient is therefore of great importance in alleviating the anxiety of admission to hospital. Few patients openly express any worries and it is therefore important to give the patient the comfort of understanding the ward environment and his part in it. The patient may feel more comfortable in the early phase in the presence of a nurse and sometimes feels more at ease talking about his condition to a male nurse.

Giving too much information at once is inadvisable, as anxiety reduces the amount retained in the memory. Many hospitals issue a pamphlet outlining the basic hospital routine prior to admission. Anxiety can manifest itself in the patient by physical signs, e.g. rapid pulse or altered blood pressure. The measures outlined are aimed purely at reducing any worry about hospital treatment.

Preoperative care and investigations

Following admission all patients have all the following investigations considered and most are performed routinely. The psychological wellbeing of the patient is vital — encouragement, reassurance and explanation of the procedure and after care are essential so the patient knows what to expect. All patients under 66 years old have the possibility of postoperative infertility explained.

1.   Full blood survey: haemoglobin, full blood count, urea and electrolytes, serum multiple analysis

2.   Serum acid phosphatase: this may be raised and indicates malignant changes

3. Group and cross-match of blood: usually two units
4. Electrocardiograph
5. Pulmonary function tests
6. Midstream specimen of urine
7. Ward test of urine
8. Intravenous pyelogram/urogram: to eliminate renal pathology or calculi formation
9. Chest X-ray
10. Weight
11. Diet: to build patient up
12. Temperature, pulse and respiration
13. Fluid balance monitoring: urine output
14. Physiotherapy: preoperative chest physiotherapy and instruction for pelvic floor exercises/bladder drill postoperatively
15. Dental check: many patients have dentures and some may need pre-or postoperative dental care
16. Rectal examination: a benign enlargement of the prostate usually has a smooth, rounded feel while a prostatic cancer has a hard, irregular outline

Immediate preoperative care
1. Routine preoperative preparation for type of anaesthesia employed
2. Pubic shave is not usually required if resection is being performed. Shaving will be required for open surgery

Suppositories, e.g. glycerine or Dulcolax, or rectal enema are required — a full bowel interferes with procedure. A finger is inserted per rectum to enhance removal of the prostate. It must be remembered that these patients are usually older and the investigations are designed to confirm diagnosis, assess renal function and provide the best possible preparation for anaesthetic. Premedication is not uncommon. Antibiotic cover is not uncommon in patients with know urinary tract infection who require surgery.

If the surgeon contemplates doing an operation to remove the prostate which will not afford a view of the bladder, e.g. retropubic (Millin) type, a cystoscopy is sometimes performed to eliminate bladder disease, e.g. calculi or tumour.

Postoperative care

Irrespective of the type of operation performed there are ten facets of postoperative care which apply and are vital to good postoperative nursing.

1. Early mobilization. These patients are predisposed to early complications. Care must be taken if epidural anaesthesia is employed. The cannula is often left in situ for 24 hours to assist postoperative analgesia. Ensure sufficient time has elapsed for numbness of the legs to have worn off. The patient is encouraged to mobilize with the catheter in situ and there is no reason why irrigation should delay this.

2. Abundant oral fluids. The patient should take at least 150-200 ml hourly. A pint or more of lager or beer is an excellent, palatable way of boosting intake and its diuretic effect helps avoid clot retention.

Fluids in large volumes should be given immediately following epidural anaesthesia or as soon as possible following general anaesthesia. Maxalon or Stemetil (anti-emetics) are often given postoperatively to prevent nausea. Intravenous therapy lines are usually left in situ until oral intake is satisfactory, usually about 18-24 hours.

3. Accurate fluid balance recording. It is the only guide to the patient's urine output (see p. 38).

4. Hematuria and clot retention. It should be remembered that the urine at the catheter end of the tube may differ completely from that in the bag. The urine should ideally be no darker than a 'rosé' wine.

5. Encouragement. Many patients worry and ask "is everything going according to plan?". Reassure the patient that the blood-stained urine is not unexpected, that the catheter will only be in situ as long as is absolutely necessary, and that the tubes will be removed as soon as possible.

6. Catheter patency. Never clamp the catheter as there is a danger of clot retention. This maintains catheter patency.

7. Fixing the catheter. Secure the catheter to prevent 'yo-yo' effect, which can introduce urinary tract infection, or precipitate haemorrhage. Care must be taken when fixing the catheter that the pressure on the meatus is avoided or it may cause a pressure sore.

8. Adequate analgesia. Adequate pain relief is essential. Usually a controlled drug, e.g., morphine 10 mg intramuscularly, is prescribed.

9. Prevent constipation. Constipation must be prevented as it can cause retention of urine or make voiding difficult post catheter removal, or cause haemorrhage, due to the patient straining to have a motion.

10. Postoperative bladder drill (see page 156). Slight urgency is not uncommon even for days postoperatively, until the bladder and bladder neck muscles regain their tone. Some patients following prostatectomy have poor bladder (detrusor) muscle function and the instillation into the bladder of prostaglandin (Prostin E2) 0.5 mg diluted in 20 ml of water has been shown in many patients to increase bladder contraction and therefore aid bladder tone. This is used mostly in patients with chronic retention (enlarged bladder) with no outflow obstruction postoperatively, but prostaglandin (Prostin E2) instillation has also been used in the treatment of patients post-hysterectomy, post-colporrhaphy and in urodynamic studies of the lower urinary tract.

Slight bleeding at the begining or at the end of the stream is not uncommon. Some discomfort can be expected but all of these problems generally resolve without treatment.

The use of a urine bottle is essential to measure urine but there are a few points regarding bottle management which need consideration. Bottles should not be issued from a bottle trolley on a bottle round as this is a potential site for cross-infection. Disposable bottles avoid the problems associated with cleaning, but bottles made of plastic or glass are used more frequently. It is better to use a urinal sterilizer, but if none is available each patient should have his own bottle which should be scalded after emptying and regularly disinfected in a chemical cleaner. Handwashing is mandatory after emptying a bottle and if the patient is known to have a urinary tract infection, hand disinfection is recommended. Some patients do not realize the risk of contracting an infection if they lie with a bottle between their legs, so this should obviously be discouraged. They often do this because they fear bedwetting, but having the bottle in bed with them does not give the patient the incentive to regain self-control.

The usual postoperative follow-up consists of an outpatient appointment, 3 months after discharge.

Some urologists like to measure urinary flow rate to assess the effect of the surgery, or a cystoscopy is performed after 3 months has elapsed. A cystoscopy is usually mandatory, if there was any suspicion of carcinoma.

Antibiotic therapy is not given as a routine, but only if infection is present or diagnosed. Any preoperative antibiotic therapy would be continued postoperatively. In order to identify any postoperative infection, a catheter specimen of urine is taken prior to catheter removal and a mid-stream specimen of urine taken post-removal, before discharging the patient.

Complications of prostatic surgery

1. Bleeding: (a) reactionary
              (b) secondary
2. Clot retention — producing severe pain, discomfort and shock
3. Renal failure — reflex anuria
4. Urine tract infection
5. Epididymo-orchitis — infection along the vas. Vasectomy at the time of surgery prevents this complication
6. Sterility — internal sphincter damage results in retrograde ejaculation. For this reason all patients under 66 years are advised at time of giving consent to surgery.
7. Incontinence — bladder drill/pelvic floor exercises/drug therapy — patient may have persistent dribbling incontinence due to sphincter damage
8. Recurrent retention — due to (a) scar tissue or flap of prostatic tissue at bladder neck or (b) not enough tissue taken
9. Error — perforated bladder or capsule (transurethral resection of prostate) — extravasation of urine
10. Bladder neck stenosis
11. Urethral stricture

Falling into the older age group these patients are also more prone to general postoperative complications e.g. chest infections, deep vein thrombosis, etc. Anti-emboli stockings are sometimes used as a prophylactic measure.

Prostatic surgery

Transurethral resection of prostate (TURP) (Figs. 11, 12 and 13) is the operation of choice if possible. It is contraindicated in a minority of cases because of great enlargement, or ankylosis of the hip preventing correct positioning in theatre.

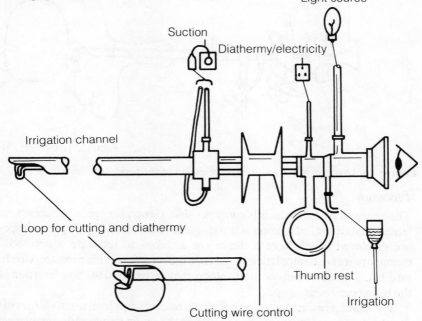

Figure 11. Diagram of a resectoscope

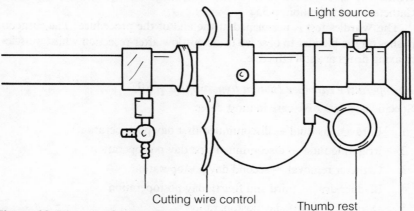

Figure 12. Diagram of a resectoscope

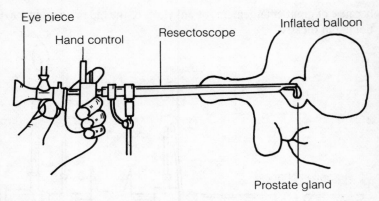

Figure 13. Diagram of a transurethral resection of the prostate

Procedure

The patient is placed in the lithotomy position. General or epidural anaesthetic is used, and controlled hypotension induced to reduce blood loss. Special drapes are employed which have a finger cot attached to facilitate a per rectal examination and manipulation to enhance the resection of the prostate. Urethral dilatation, meatotomy or urethrotomy may be required to allow insertion of the wide bore resectoscope.

The gland is resected using a specialized resectoscope loop to cut slithers off the gland. Haemostasis is achieved by using the resectoscope with coagulation diathermy. Good vision is maintained by the use of irrigation fluid (see Catheters and irrigation, p 35)

The Wardles test is performed at the end of the procedure. The surgeon pushes on the bladder to observe urine outflow after resection whilst muscle-relaxing drugs are still effective.

Postoperative care (see Benign hypertrophy, p 80)

Specific postoperative care in most cases:

1. Intravenous fluid — discontinued first day postoperation
2. Irrigating fluid — discontinued first day postoperation
3. Catheter removal — second day postoperation
4. Bladder drill — third and fourth day postoperation
5. Discharge — fifth day postoperation

In some cases diuresis may be induced rather than postoperative irrigation to flush the catheter/bleeding and each surgeon has a regime of preference

Drug therapy

1. Frusemide (Lasix),40 mg intravenous — theatre
2. Hartmans solution 1 litre intravenous — 6 hours
3. Frusemide (Lasix,) 40 mg intravenous — 3 hours postoperative
4. 5% dextrose, one litre — 12 hourly

Retropubic (Millin's) prostatectomy

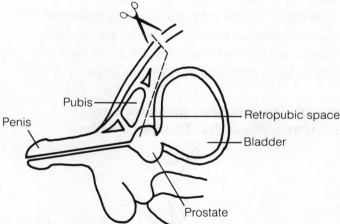

Penis

Pubis

Retropubic space

Bladder

Prostate

Figure 14. Diagram to show open prostatectomy — retropubic prostatectomy

Retropubic prostatectomy is an operation to remove the enlarged glandular tissue by exposing the capsule (the outer covering) of the prostate gland, making an incision and removing the tissue through that incision. The operation is used if transurethral resection of prostate is contraindicated or if there is no bladder condition requiring surgical treatment at the time of operation.

Procedure
The patient is placed with his head slightly down to prevent intestines obscuring or interfering with the operation. General anaesthesia is used.

A transverse skin incision is made to expose and open the prostatic capusle. The glands are enucleated with the finger, and any calculi in the bladder are removed by opening the bladder neck. Bleeding is stopped with diathermy. The capsule is sutured, and a 3-way simplastic catheter passed. Irrigation is commenced to prevent clot retention. A Redivac drain is inserted above the prostate capsule and the skin is sutured.

Postoperative care (see Benign hypertrophy, p 80)Specific postoperative care includes:

1. The patient is mobilized as soon as tolerated
2. Redivac suction released after 24 hours
3. Redivac drain removed after 48 hours (if there is any fluid collection, the drain can be left in situ until it subsides)
4. Irrigating fluid taken down 2nd or 3rd day postoperation
5. Catheter taken out about 4th or 5th day postoperation
6. Bladder drill practised from 5th or 6th day onward
7. The patient is discharged when surgeon prefers.

Suprapubic (transvesical) prostatectomy
Freyers, Harris, Wilson Hey, Thompsom Walker

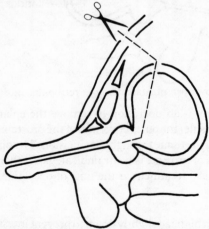

Figure 15. Diagram to show open prostatectomy — transvesical prostatectomy

Suprapubic prostatectomy is rarely used. It is the removal of the prostate gland by exposing and opening the bladder and removing the prostate through the bladder neck. It is employed if there is any bladder condition requiring surgical treatment, as well as the prostatic removal.

Procedure

The patient is placed in the Trendelenburg (head down tilt) position, and a general anaesthetic is administered. A transverse skin incision is made to expose and open the bladder. Surgery to the bladder is performed. A finger is inserted through the bladder neck and the gland is enucleated. Diathermy is sometimes used to enhance removal. Bleeding is stopped by diathermy, and a 3-way simplastic catheter is passed. The bladder is sewn up. Irrigation to prevent clot retention is commenced. A Redivac drain is inserted, and the skin sutured.

Postoperative care

As for retropubic prostatectomy, although a catheter may be left in situ slightly longer (from 7-10 days). The drain may be left in situ until after the catheter is removed and remains for a further 24-48 hours to prevent urine collection in the abdomen, if there is any extravasation of urine through the bladder suture line.

Carcinoma of prostate

Carcinoma of the prostate is a fairly common condition seen in middle aged and older men. It is affected by the sex hormones and their production alters carcinoma growth, e.g. testosterone (male hormone) stimulates growth, oestrogen (female hormone) inhibits growth. Adenocarcinoma (carcinoma affecting glandular tissue) is the most usual form.

Causes

The causes are unknown. It often spreads

1. Directly or locally into the bladder and may involve the ureters
2. Via the lymphatic system
3. Via the blood. Bone and lung are common deposit sites.

Signs and symptoms

The signs and symptoms are similar to those for benign hypertrophy. Many cases are found on histology following resection for enlarged prostate. Due to the nature of the disease, it may produce symptoms associated with carcinoma changes from secondary deposits, e.g. cough, alteration to bowel habit, lassitude, malaise, back pain and oedema of the legs.

Investigations

As for benign hypertrophy, and

1. Per rectal examination — the tumour feels irregular and hard

2. Blood examination — low haemoglobin leading to anaemia associated with metastasis; elevated urea indicates renal impairment; high serum acid phosphatase is suggestive of carcinoma (the normal prostate secretes a small amount)

3. Radiological examination — skeletal survey and bone scan to show secondary deposits, risk of pathological facture); chest X-ray to eliminate secondary lung deposits

4. Cystoscopy to eliminate bladder involvement

5. Urine cytology to demonstrate malignant cells in urine

6. Biopsy taken with a biopsy needle e.g. Trucut. The patient lies on his side. The surgeon, using his finger as a guide, advances the needle and takes the biopsy via the rectum. Prophylactic antibiotic therapy is often employed with this technique (tobramycin 120 mg intramuscular stat. given pre-procedure and trimethoprim (Ipral) 200 mg orally twice daily given for 3 days post biopsy). The biopsy may be obtained by perineal stab under local anaesthetic. An aseptic technique is employed with the patient lying in lithotomy position. This method is used less frequently than the rectal technique.

Treatment

Treatment can vary, but usually consists of

1. Hormone therapy

2. Transurethral resection of prostate tumour

3. Radiotherapy

4. Sub capsular orchidectomy

Hormone therapy. Although used less frequently than previously, hormone therapy is used to alter the body hormone levels aimed at suppressing prostatic carcinoma changes. Examples of therapies are:

Stilboesterol 1 mg tablets 1-3 mg daily (a higher loading dose is often given to initiate therapy);

Fosfestrol tetrasodium, a synthetic oestrogen (Honvan) 276 mg injection 2-4 ampoules (5 ml of 55.2 mg/ml) for 5 days with 2-4 ampoules weekly follow up. This injection does carry some initial side effects. Pain in the perineum can be quite severe and a pre-medication of papaveretum (Omnopon) intramuscular injection is often prescribed. Nausea following injection of Honvan is not uncommon and can be quite marked requiring anti-emetic therapy. Intravenous chlorpromazine (Largactil) is sometimes given in conjunction with this drug.

Honvan is used more often than stilboesterol usually after sub-capsular orchidectomy.

Transurethral resection of prostate tumour. Usually a transurethral resection, as for benign prostatic hypertrophy, is performed to allow the patient to pass urine better. Pre- and postoperative care is identical to transurethral resection of prostate.

Radiotherapy. Radiotherapy is not usually used as a curative procedure but more often as a follow-up treatment following resection.

Subcapsular orchidectomy. Subcapsular orchidectomy to remove the glandular tissue is performed in the treatment of prostatic carcinoma in preference to stilboesterol (hormone) therapy. It reduces the male hormone production which affects the prostatic growth and helps control the pain from metastasis. It is usually performed after transurethral resection (see orchidectomy, p 62).

Further reading

Blacklock N J (1979) Prostatitis, Practitioner 223 (1335): 318-22

Blandy J P (1976) Benign enlargement of the prostate, Nursing Mirror 143 (9): 47-51

Bridges N (1980) Transurethral resection of the benign enlarged prostate, (Theatre Nursing Care Study), Nursing Times 76 (48): 2098-2107

Chartham R (1982) Ante- and post-prostatectomy supportive therapy (impotence), Practitioner 226 (1373):1965-1967

Cranston J A (1978) Benign enlargement of the prostate gland, Nursing Times 74 (19): 789-794

Datta P K (1981a) Prostatic patient, bladder and neck obstruction, Nursing Times 77 (40): 1717-1718

Datta P K (1981b) Post-prostatectomy patient, Nursing Times 77 (41): 175-1761

Hadfield J (1981) When once is not enough, Clinical Forum, urological emergencies, Nursing Mirror 152 (4) supplt

Iveson-Iveson J (1980) Acute urine retention (Long answer question), students forum, Nursing Mirror 150 (9): 25-26

Iveson-Iveson J (1982) Enlarged prostate, students forum, Nursing Mirror 154 (3): 32

Jameson R M (1982) Impotence and prostatectomy, Practitioner 226 (1373): 1969

Main J M (1978) Prostatitis, Nursing Times 74 (19): 787-788

Molitor P (1983) Transurethral resection, Nursing Mirror 157 (14): 22-27

Parson A A (1981) A patient with benign prostate hyperplasia, (pre and postoperative care), Nursing Times : 1081-1083

Smart J Gordon (1979) Carcinoma of the prostate, Practitioner 223 (1335): 312-317

Smith P (1978) Prostatic and bladder neck syndrome I, Nursing Times 74 (23): 956-960

Twinham J (1980) Transurethral resection of prostate (Nursing Care Study), Nursing Times 76 (48): 2094-2097

CHAPTER 7

BLADDER ABNORMALITIES

There are various bladder abnormalities, but two important conditions are diverticulum and bladder neck obstruction.

Bladder diverticulum

Bladder diverticulum, as a congenital abnormality, is rare but can occur if the bladder outlet is obstructed.

Signs and symptoms

The signs and symptoms usually reflect the problems of urine stasis including repeated urinary tract infection, and bladder calculi formation

Investigation/diagnosis

1. Intravenous pyelogram
2. Cystoscopy

Treatment

Treatment is two fold: to relieve any bladder outlet obstruction, and to remove the sac (diverticulectomy.)

Preoperatve preparation. As for open prostatectomy

Postoperative care

1. As for open prostatectomy
2. Wound drainage via Redivac drainage for 3-4 days (suction may be released after 24 hours)

Bladder neck obstruction

Increased fibrous tissue of the bladder neck, reducing the opening, can occur at any age. The danger of this condition is the risk to the upper urinary tract caused by back pressure of urine over a long period.

Signs and symptoms

1. Poor stream
2. Dribbling
3. Repeated urinary tract infection

Investigation/diagnosis

1. Intravenous pyelogram
2. Cystoscopy
3. Cystometry
4. Patients age — patients are often too young for symptoms to be due to prostatic disease

Treatment

Treatment is transurethral resection of bladder neck. From 1-4 incisions into the outlet are made to allow a free flow.

Pre-and postoperative care. Identical to transurethral resection of prostate.

Cystitis

Cystitis is an inflammation of the lining of the bladder. It is very common, occuring more frequently in women that in men, due to the anatomical structure in the female. It is most often due to bacterial infection with *E. coli*, which can reach the bladder from:

1. Urethra — by catheterization or instrumentation
    — from existing urethral infection
    — venereal disease
2. Kidney — descending infection.

Many factors predispose to the condition:

1. Urine retention
2. Existing infection, e.g. urethritis, prostatitis
3. Debilitating disease
4. Diabetes mellitus
5. Pregnancy
6. Trauma (catheters, etc.)
7. Sexual intercourse (honeymoon cystitis)
8. Vaginitis, vulvitis

Signs and symptoms

1. Suprapubic pain
2. Frequency
3. Buring and scalding sensation on micturition. Worse in the morning and improves as fluids are taken
4. Tenderness in suprapubic region, often with associated dull ache in lower abdomen
5. Passing only small amounts of urine
6. Blood in urine
7. Strong or offensive smelling urine

Investigations

1. Midstream specimen of urine (early morning specimen if tuberculosis is suspected
2. Ward test of urine (cloudy, smelly, pus, blood)
3. Cystoscopy — more for investigation for chronic cystitis

Treatment

Treatment is aimed at preventing recurrent attacks. Four main areas are considered:

1. Personal hygiene
2. Sexual activity

3.   Diet
4.   Fluid intake.

Personal hygiene. After a bowel motion, skin should be gently cleaned from front to back with soft tissue. The vaginal and anal area should be washed with a soapy flannel, rinsed and dried. The flannel should be used for that purpose only and boiled at least once a week. Underclothes should be changed at least once a day and cotton underwear worn, as opposed to nylon. Cosmetics, e.g. vaginal deodorants, bath oils, bubble baths, talcum powder, should be avoided. Any vaginal discharge must investigated.

Sexual activity. Both partners should shower, bath or wash before intercourse. The foreskin should be retracted before washing (if not circumcised). Lubricants should be used to prevent soreness or bruising. The bladder should be emptied within 30 minutes following intercourse (to wash out any bacteria that may have entered the urethra).

Diet. Fibre content of the diet should be increased, and surplus refined sugar and starches avoided (to prevent excessive accumulation of bacteria in the bowel) . Foods containing refined sugar and white, refined flour, e.g. sugar, sweets, jams, soft drinks, white bread and cakes, should also be avoided. Alternatives include wholemeal flour and fresh fruit. The increased fibre intake will help to prevent constipation.

Fluid intake. Fluid intake should be enough to maintain a daily output of at least 8—9 litres. If an attack is starting, fluid intake should consist of:

1.   A pint of fluid every half hour, (water, weak tea, diluted flavoured drinks). Barley water is often recommended without any real reason. It is best to avoid strong tea or coffee.
2.   Drinking until retiring to bed at night and taking further fluid when waking to pass urine.
     Alcoholic drink may be taken in moderation provided other fluids are continued.

Drugs. Bladder relaxants may be prescribed, e.g. emepronium bromide (Cetiprin) may be given for bladder spasm due to infection. Potassium citrate mixture may be given to ease cystitis symptoms, e.g. scalding sensation.

Sodium bicarbonate is sometimes given to reduce the acidity of the urine and to help relieve the burning sensation in acute episodes. Care is taken to ensure that there is no renal impairment before employing or advising this treatment, as it carries a risk of causing alkalosis.

Antibiotic therapy may be prescribed and is given for 3—10 days. If the patient has difficulty remembering to take tablets, suitable drugs are employed which can be taken twice or at most three times a day.

Rest and warmth. Sometimes a hot water bottle over the abdomen or between the thighs helps to relieve the pain.

Education. Encourage the patient to learn more about cystitis and its associated conditions by reading material available from the Health Education Council and "Self Help in Cystitis" and "Understanding Cystitis" available from the U and I Club, (See p.110).

Complications

Chronic cystitis, invariably due to some underlying disease.

Neurogenic bladder

Neurogenic bladder is the term used to describe a disturbance of bladder function by interference or interruption to its nerve supply. This may occur at the level of the spinal cord or higher (including the brain).

Trauma, neoplasm, inflammatory or degenerative changes about the level of the spinal cord reflex arc controlling the bladder will result in a totally automatic function with no or decreased higher centre control. Injury or lesion of the spinal cord or peripheral nerves destroys the reflex impulses. This destroys the normal voiding impulses, and urine is released as overflow.

Signs and symptoms

Disturbance to normal pattern of micturition.

Investigations

1. Physical examination
2. Intravenous pyelogram
3. Cystometry
4. Cysto-urethroscopy

Treatment

Treatment is related to the underlying cause, e.g. spinal injury. Urological treatment is aimed at avoiding complications, e.g. manual compression emptying of bladder; catheterization.

Complications

1. Repeated urinary tract infection
2. Chronic infection of urinary tree and kidneys
3. Renal failure

Bladder trauma

The bladder is commonly injured as a result of multiple injury, but injury may occur as a result of surgery close to the bladder e.g. hysterectomy. The bladder is susceptible to injury during endoscopic procedures, especially if a transurethral resection of bladder tumour is being performed. A distended bladder is more vulnerable to injury.

Signs and symptoms

Urine will leak into the body tissue in the vicinity of the urinary tract (extravasation of urine). This is shown by:

General symptoms	Local symptoms
1. Shock — low blood pressure — circulatory failure	1. Paralytic ileus
	2. peritonitis — rigidity of abdominal wall
2. Raised temperature	3. Perineal bruising
	4. Urethral bleeding
	5. Swollen perineum
	6. No urine output

Investigations

1. History — physical examination or recent history and procedure suggests injury

2. General appearance
3. X-ray of pelvis (fracture)
4. Intravenous pyelogram
5. Cystogram
6. Haemoglobin
7. Cross match blood

Treatment

1. Treat the patient for shock
2. Repair tear — insert a suprapubic catheter if tear is large or near urethra.
3. Drain wound for up to 5 days (some surgeons leave drain until the catheter has been removed)
4. Catheterize the patient for up to 7 days

Complications

1. Infection, e.g. pelvic, bladder, renal, peritonitis
2. Paralytic ileus
3. Fistula
4. Haemorrhage
5. Bladder neck stenosis

Bladder fistulae

Bladder fistulae are rare but tend to be more common in females.

Causes

1. Neoplasm, e.g. of bladder, bowel, female reproductive tract
2. Postoperative complication, e.g. after transurethral resection of tumour.
3. Post-radiotherapy, e.g. of cervix
4. Trauma

Signs and symptoms

Vaginal fistula	**Bowel fistula** (this may also be as a result of diverticular disease)
1. Persistent incontinence	1. Pneumaturia (passing air as well as urine)
2. Generally unwell (malaise, sweating, etc)	2. Faeces in urine

Diagnosis

1. Physical examination	1. Physical examination
2. Intravenous pyelogram	2. Predisposing history e.g. diverticulitis
3. Mid-stream specimen of urine	3. Barium enema
4. Cystoscopy	4. Sigmoidoscopy

Treatment

1. Repair vaginal fistula and bladder wall	1. Repair bladder fistula
2. Catheterize patient for 7 - 14 days	2. Resection of diseased bowel
3. Repeated mid-stream specimens of urine (to observe for and treat infection rapidly)	3. Temporary colostomy

Complications

1. Haematuria
2. Infection
3. Failure to heal (second repair required)

Bladder neoplasm

The treatment of cancer of the urological system, particularly the bladder, is a major part of the work of the urologist. Most cancers of the bladder originate from its epithelial lining, but may also be as a result of invasion from other sites e.g. bowel. Bladder cancer is more common in men than in women. (about 3:1) and it affects generally the older age group (60-70 years).

Causes

Although the causes are unknown, predisposing factors include:

1. Chronic cystitis
2. Bladder diverticula
3. Exposure to carcinogenic chemicals, e.g. synthetic rubber (many firms insist upon regular medical checks for employees)
4. Smoking
5. Calculi

Cancer of the bladder can affect any area of the bladder but it often affects the base of the bladder (including the bladder exit) and ureteric orifices.

Types of cancer

Benign cancer (papilloma) of the bladder is uncommon. Cancer tends to be malignant and the type of growths include:

1. Differentiated transitional cell carcinoma — tend to be smaller tumours with little invasive tendency and are usually like a cauliflower (papillary) in appearance.
2. Undifferentiated transitional cell carcinoma — a more invasive type of carcinoma with generally a very irregular growth, more wart-or ulcer-like in appearance.
3. Squamous cell carcinoma — an invasive type of cancer which tends to be bulky.
4. Adenocarcinoma — a less common form of cancer affecting the base of the bladder

Grading. A grading system is used to describe the extent of a growth:

1. Direct — stage one (TI), confined to the inner lining (urothelium) of

bladder only
— stage two (T2), into muscle (but less than half way through)
— stage three (T3), into muscle (over half way through)
— stage four (T4), eroded through bladder.

The diagnosis of T2 and T3 tumours is difficult and it is the surgeon's experience together with the biopsy results which enables the grade to be assessed.

2.   Lymphatic spread — usually via the groin nodes, the area in grade three tumours is rich in lymphatics.
3.   Blood borne spread — usually a late development resulting in secondary deposits, e.g. in lung, liver, bone.
4.   Implantation — e.g. into prostatic bed, urethra or remaining bladder wall.

Signs and symptoms
The signs and symptoms vary in degree and number and may include:

1.   Haematuria — fresh and painless (single most common symptom of bladder cancer). Most patients seeking advice present with painless haematuria. In later stages clots may develop.
2.   Infection, cystitis, pyelonephritis
3.   Ureteric obstruction, hydronephrosis, pyelonephritis
4.   Urethral obstruction, poor stream, frequency
5.   Direct spread
6.   Fistula formation
7.   Dribbling incontinence
8.   Pain
9.   Palpable tumour.

Investigations
1.   Abdominal X-ray
2.   Chest X-ray — to investigate for lung metastasis
3.   Cystogram
4.   Per rectal examination

SEFTON GENERAL HOSPITAL

DEPARTMENT OF UROLOGY
PAPILLOMA CLINIC

PATIENT IDENTIFYING DETAILS (ADDRESSOGRAM)

AGE	NAME GROUP	RADIOTHERAPY No.

FAMILY HISTORY

DIAGNOSIS	YEAR

OCCUPATION

HISTORY	DURATION (in weeks)

PYELOGRAM (At least every two years)

Date	Report

RADIOTHERAPY

Date	Dose	Duration

DATE

ORIGINAL TUMOUR

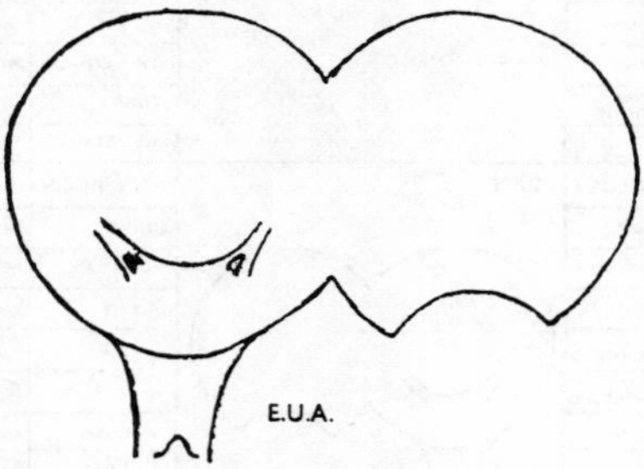

DESCRIPTION		
SINGLE		
MULTIPLE		
SIZE (CMS.)	<3	
	3-5	
	> 5	
MUCOSAL		
MUSCLE—SUPERFICIAL		
MUSCLE—DEEP		
EXTRAVESICAL		
FIXED		
METASTASES		

HISTOLOGY	
PAPILLARY	
MIXED	
SOLID	
WELL DIFFERENTIA'D	
POORLY DIFFERENTIA'D	
ANAPLASTIC	
NO INVASION	
INVASION	
METAPLASIA	
SARCOMA AND OTHER	

FIRST TREATMENT		
SURGICAL	Fulguration	
	T.U.R.	
	Suprapubic Excision	
	Partial Cystectomy	
	Total Cystectomy	
	Other	
Radio Therapy	Inter Stitial	
	H.E.R.	
Chemo Therapy	Local	
	General	
OTHER		
DIAGNOSIS ONLY		
INOPERABLE		
PALLIATIVE ONLY		
COMPLICATIONS		

MED/C 335.61 1.76

Figure 16. Chart to show cystoscopy results

DATE

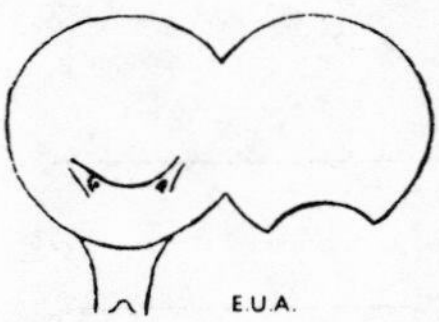

E.U.A.

TREATMENT

DESCRIPTION		HISTOLOGY
SINGLE		PAPILLARY
MULTIPLE		MIXED
SIZE (CMS.)	<3	SOLID
	3-5	WELL DIFFERENTIA'D
	> 5	POORLY DIFFERENTIA'D
MUCOSAL		ANAPLASTIC
MUSCLE—SUPERFICIAL		NO INVASION
MUSCLE—DEEP		INVASION
EXTRAVESICAL		METAPLASIA
FIXED		SARCOMA AND OTHER
METASTASES		

DATE

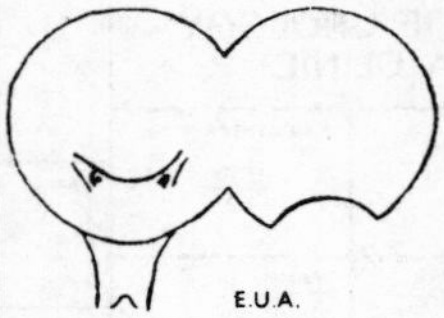

E.U.A.

TREATMENT

DESCRIPTION		HISTOLOGY
SINGLE		PAPILLARY
MULTIPLE		MIXED
SIZE (CMS.)	<3	SOLID
	3-5	WELL DIFFERENTIA'D
	> 5	POORLY DIFFERENTIA'D
MUCOSAL		ANAPLASTIC
MUSCLE—SUPERFICIAL		NO INVASION
MUSCLE—DEEP		INVASION
EXTRAVESICAL		METAPLASIA
FIXED		SARCOMA AND OTHER
METASTASES		

DATE

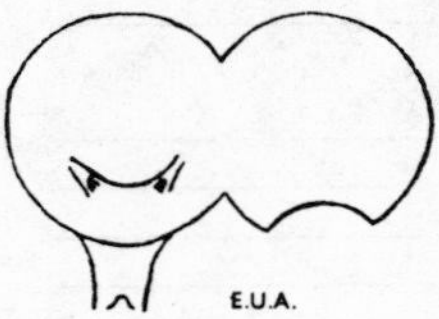

E.U.A.

TREATMENT

DESCRIPTION		HISTOLOGY
SINGLE		PAPILLARY
MULTIPLE		MIXED
SIZE (CMS.)	<3	SOLID
	3-5	WELL DIFFERENTIA'D
	> 5	POORLY DIFFERENTIA'D
MUCOSAL		ANAPLASTIC
MUSCLE—SUPERFICIAL		NO INVASION
MUSCLE—DEEP		INVASION
EXTRAVESICAL		METAPLASIA
FIXED		SARCOMA AND OTHER
METASTASES		

DATE

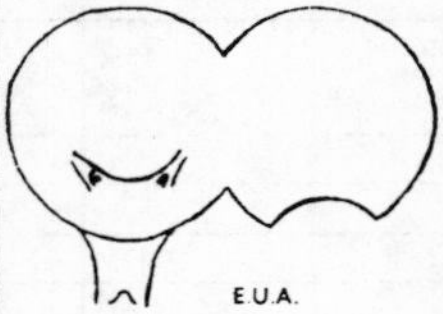

E.U.A.

TREATMENT

DESCRIPTION		HISTOLOGY
SINGLE		PAPILLARY
MULTIPLE		MIXED
SIZE (CMS.)	<3	SOLID
	3-5	WELL DIFFERENTIA'D
	> 5	POORLY DIFFERENTIA'D
MUCOSAL		ANAPLASTIC
MUSCLE—SUPERFICIAL		NO INVASION
MUSCLE—DEEP		INVASION
EXTRAVESICAL		METAPLASIA
FIXED		SARCOMA AND OTHER
METASTASES		

DATE

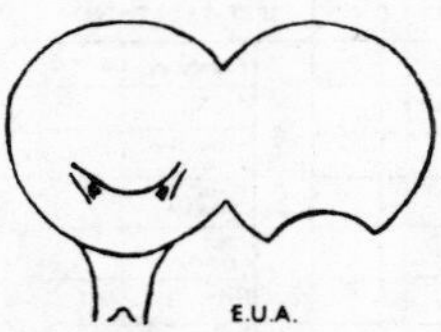

E.U.A.

TREATMENT

DESCRIPTION		HISTOLOGY
SINGLE		PAPILLARY
MULTIPLE		MIXED
SIZE (CMS.)	<3	SOLID
	3-5	WELL DIFFERENTIA'D
	> 5	POORLY DIFFERENTIA'D
MUCOSAL		ANAPLASTIC
MUSCLE—SUPERFICIAL		NO INVASION
MUSCLE—DEEP		INVASION
EXTRAVESICAL		METAPLASIA
FIXED		SARCOMA AND OTHER
METASTASES		

DATE

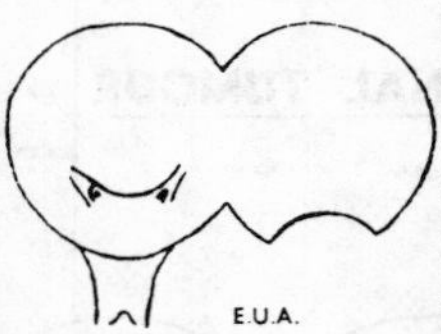

E.U.A.

TREATMENT

DESCRIPTION		HISTOLOGY
SINGLE		PAPILLARY
MULTIPLE		MIXED
SIZE (CMS.)	<3	SOLID
	3-5	WELL DIFFERENTIA'D
	> 5	POORLY DIFFERENTIA'D
MUCOSAL		ANAPLASTIC
MUSCLE—SUPERFICIAL		NO INVASION
MUSCLE—DEEP		INVASION
EXTRAVESICAL		METAPLASIA
FIXED		SARCOMA AND OTHER
METASTASES		

DATE

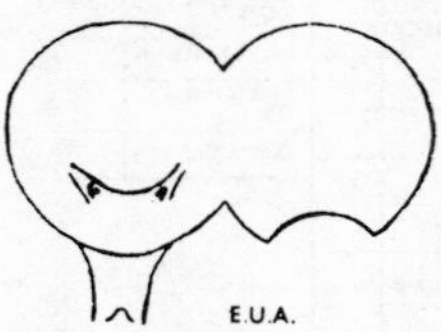

E.U.A.

TREATMENT

DESCRIPTION		HISTOLOGY
SINGLE		PAPILLARY
MULTIPLE		MIXED
SIZE (CMS.)	<3	SOLID
	3-5	WELL DIFFERENTIA'D
	> 5	POORLY DIFFERENTIA'D
MUCOSAL		ANAPLASTIC
MUSCLE—SUPERFICIAL		NO INVASION
MUSCLE—DEEP		INVASION
EXTRAVESICAL		METAPLASIA
FIXED		SARCOMA AND OTHER
METASTASES		

DATE

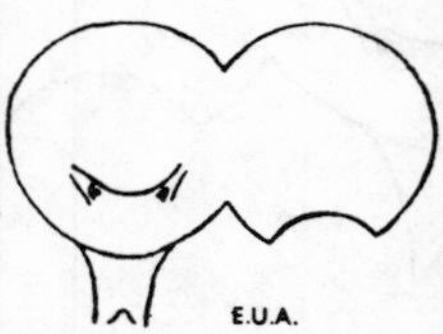

E.U.A.

TREATMENT

DESCRIPTION		HISTOLOGY
SINGLE		PAPILLARY
MULTIPLE		MIXED
SIZE (CMS.)	<3	SOLID
	3-5	WELL DIFFERENTIA'D
	> 5	POORLY DIFFERENTIA'D
MUCOSAL		ANAPLASTIC
MUSCLE—SUPERFICIAL		NO INVASION
MUSCLE—DEEP		INVASION
EXTRAVESICAL		METAPLASIA
FIXED		SARCOMA AND OTHER
METASTASES		

5. Ward test of urine isolates particularly microscopic haematuria
6. Mid-stream specimen of urine
7. Bone scan — shows bone deposits and renal disease as the kidneys are highlighted during excretion of the isotope.
8. Ultrasound scan — to determine size of a fixed mass
9. Urine cytology
10. Cystoscopy — is a mandatory examination with the results often displayed on a special chart in the case sheet. (Fig. 16) The general practitioner is kept informed by means of a specially graded letter (Fig. 17).

Biopsy results are important but the grading the laboratory gives is only a guide, because the specimen depends upon the depth to which the surgeon cuts to obtain the specimen. Instead of grading the tumour T1, T2, T3 or T4, a pathologist will grade it P1, P2, P3, or P4. The combined results are used as a guide to the true extent of the tumour in the T scale. (p.99).

Treatment

The treatment of bladder cancer depends upon its grade. Cigarette smoking should be discouraged from the outset.

T1 tumours

Small tumours, providing they are not numerous, are destroyed by burning (diathermy, fulguration) following biopsy. If tumours are present in great numbers, making diathermy impracticable, bladder instillations of cytotoxic drugs are used e.g. ethoglucid (Epodyl) and doxyrubicin (Adriamycin).

Bladder tumours in numbers not allowing therapy may be treated by the use of Helmstein's balloon therapy. As a final resort if these measures are not applicable or are unsucessful, removal of the bladder may be required (cystectomy).

Cystoscopy/cystodiathermy are usually performed under general anaesthesia, though epidural anaesthesia may be used.

Preoperative preparation consists of preparing the patient for general anaesthesia. A pubic shave is not required.

Postoperatively, encourage the patient to take oral fluids as soon as possible after surgery. Urine output is monitored carefully noting the depth of haematuria and the volume of urine.

Dear Dr.   Re:—

Your patient underwent a check cyctoscopy as follow up for bladder carcinoma on

CYSTOSCOPY REVEALED

☐ 1) No sign of recurrent tumour

☐ 2) Superficial tumour recurrences   ☐ Minor

☐ 3) Radiotherapy changes   ☐ Extensive

☐ 4) Evidence of muscle invasion   ☐ Local

☐ 5) Spread beyond bladder   ☐ Distant metastases

TREATMENT

☐ 1) None required

☐ 2) Transurethral resection/Fulguration

☐ 3) Biopsy

☐ 4) Other

FURTHER MANAGEMENT

☐ 1) Check cyctoscopy in   months   ☐ In-patient

☐ 2) Urine cytology as outpatient   ☐ Day case

☐ 3) Referral for radiotherapy

☐ 4) Intravesical cytotoxic drugs

☐ 5) Review in outpatients

☐ 6) Readmission for surgery

Figure 17. Example of letter to general practitioner to show cystoscopy results

A catheter is not always left in situ postoperatively and if one is, it is generally removed within 24 hours of surgery. The patient usually remains in hospital overnight but the overall duration as an inpatient depends upon urine output, urinary control, haematuria (in any depth), and the presence of infection requiring treatment.

Bladder instillations of cytotoxic drugs. The aim of cytotoxic bladder instillations is to bring the cytotoxic drug into direct contact with diseased bladder surface. A course of bladder instillations, often over a 6-month period, is followed by cystoscopy to assess its effectiveness. The patient usually attends the urological ward once a month for 6 months for the bladder instillation. In some cases the surgeon intensifies the course to six weekly instillations followed by cystoscopy. The hospital policy for the preparation of cytotoxic drugs is followed.

NOTE: Many cytotoxic anticancer drugs carry hazards, from being mutagenic to the possibility of being carcinogenic. It is vital therefore that handling, preparation and administration of these drugs be performed with the utmost care.

Administration of cytotoxic drugs

1.   Whenever possible have the hospital pharmacy prepare the instillation

2.   Wear at least a long sleeved gown/apron and mask, and protect the eyes.

3.   Wear protective gloves of PVC

4.   Work on double thickness paper towels to contain spillage

5.   Open ampoules using fibre-free sterile towel or sterile alcohol wipe

6.   Use luer lock closures when possible

7.   Avoid generating pressure in rubber-capped vials by introducing diluant slowly, allowing dispelled air to bubble back into the syringe

8.   Excess air or drug in a syringe should be expelled into a sterile towel

9.   All sharps (needles, ampoules) should go into a separate rigid container reserved for cytotoxic waste

10. All other waste should go into two polythene bags, one inside the other and should be burned without opening. The bags should be clearly labelled to stress the point.

General precautions

1. Do not handle cytotoxic drugs if pregnant
2. Any spillage should be cleaned with paper towels and mopped with large amounts of soap and water
3. If anything is spilled onto skin, wash it off with large amounts of water. Eye contamination should be irrigated with large volumes of normal saline 0.9%. Medical advice should always be sought.

Procedure The patient is catheterized and the reconstituted drug is carefully instilled into the bladder avoiding any skin contamination. Normal saline is usually used to reconstitute the drugs, and some drugs (e.g. ethoglucid, Epodyl) need to be given with a glass syringe.

Fluid intake should be reduced 12 hours pre-instillation, so that the urine volume is reduced. The catheter is usually clamped and the solution retained in the bladder for 45-60 minutes.

Whilst the fluid is in the bladder, the patient should be instructed to turn to different positions — front, both sides and back — usually for about 10 minutes to ensure that the total bladder surface is exposed to the drug.

Some patients find it easier to tolerate the solution if the catheter is removed, but if the catheter is left in situ during instillation, it is removed at the completion of treatment without draining the solution so that the urethra is exposed to the drug during micturition.

Cytotoxic drugs do affect the normal bladder cells and can therefore cause the bladder to have less capacity than is usual with a resultant frequency of urine. Drugs used in cytotoxic bladder instillation include:

1. Doxurobicin (Adriamycin) from 50 mg but usually 80 mg in 100 ml saline solution
2. Ethoglucid (Epodyl) 1% solution
3. Formalin.

Helmstein's balloon therapy. The aim of Helmstein's balloon therapy is to cause necrosis of the projecting tumour growths in the bladder, by pressure from a balloon inflated on a Helmstein's balloon catheter. Usually performed in theatre, the procedure is quite long, and the catheter being left in situ for a long time. In some hospitals this procedure is done with the patient heavily sedated, and the patient is nursed on the ward with observations recorded every 15 minutes.

Oral fluids are encouraged after this procedure. A catheter is left in situ following treatment (the urine often has a very strong aroma following this procedure).

T2 tumours

T2 tumours are usually treated by transurethral resection of tumour. A diathermy cutting loop is used to remove the tissue. The pre- and postoperative care are similar to the care for urethral resection of prostate. (p.80).

T3 tumours

Radiotherapy may be considered for these patients, but often some form of surgical removal is necessary, as it may for multiple T1 or T2 tumours.

T4 tumours

T4 tumours are generally so advanced as to be inoperable with radical surgery. They are treated usually with radiotherapy. Surgery would only be undertaken to provide a palliative by-pass if ureters were obstructed.

Cystectomy

Cystectomy is the removal of the bladder. It is usually performed in cases of cancer.

Partial cystectomy. The removal of part of the bladder is used mainly in older people with a shorter life expectancy who need relief of symptoms. This avoids a more extensive major operation.

The procedure has better results if the patient has a tumour with well-defined limits.

Simple cystectomy. Simple cystectomy involves the removal of the bladder, prostate, seminal vesicles and lymph nodes. Surrounding organs and the urethra may be removed in cases of more extensive carcinoma.

Palliative surgery is sometimes performed if infiltration is extensive.

As a result of surgery the patient wll loose normal sexual capabilities due to nerve damage. Sexual counselling is therefore a necessary part of the patient's total care.

Pre- and postoperative care as for urinary diversion.

Terminal care

Patients suffering from cancer do not always respond to, or are amenable to treatment and therefore the terminal care of these patients is of great importance. Unfortunately the illness is often protracted and although many patients want to stay at home, hospital admission may be required if circumstances dictate, e.g. the patient becomes very ill, confused, persistently and unmanageably incontinent, or family circumstances intervene in their care at home. This should not preclude relatives from being involved in patient care.

Important aspects in the care of these patients must include:

1. The relief of pain. Analgesia must be adjusted and given to provide adequate pain relief. Suffering is not justified in any form. Controlled drugs are usually required e.g. dipipanone hydrochloride (Diconal) tablets, diamorphine, elixir or injection. Pain may be exacerbated by worry, apprehension and fear of the unknown.

2. The establishment of a good rapport between patient, relatives, nursing and medical teams.

3. Having a ready ear to listen and discuss the patient's condition with the patient and his obviously anxious relatives.

4. Involving the social worker in helping the patient and relatives to cope with any personal or domestic problems arising from the patient's admission.

5. The quick and individual treatment for any more distressing symptoms which may develop from the condition, e.g. vomiting, general malaise/weakness, urinary problems (debris, infection, haematuria, dehydration), painful joints/movement (with secondary bone deposits), fungating ulcers.

6. The provision for spiritual needs, encouragement in self-help and maintaining interests and hobbies. It is always preferable for the patient to be prepared for the eventual outcome and for the relatives to be present at the time of death.

Useful address
U and I Club
9e Compton Road
London N1 2PA.
(Tel: 01-359 0403)

CHAPTER 8

URINARY DIVERSIONS

Urinary diversion is the alteration of the normal path of urine outflow. The indications include any disease causing irreparable damage to pelvic region and its organs, e.g. neurological disease (spinal damage), severest forms of incontinence, gynaecological cancer, congenital conditions.

Urinary sigmoidostomy
Urinary sigmoidostomy is the implanting of ureters into the sigmoid colon. The urine is then passed per rectum. It is rarely performed now except in cases of carcinoma of the bladder.

Preoperative care
1. It is important to ensure that the patient can tolerate fluid per rectum and for some days preoperatively, retention enemas of saline are instilled in increasing quantities for an increasing length of time.

   For this reason the patient's suitability for this type of surgery must be evaluated. Important factors to consider include age, good general health, normal renal function, normal anal sphincter.

2. Pubic and perineal shave

3. Extensive bowel evacuation is necessary to reduce risk of infection. This is commenced at least 2 - 3days preoperatively. A low residue or fluids only diet is given for 48 hours preoperatively.

4. Drug therapy preoperatively to sterilize the bowel may include

   Phthalyesulphathiazole — 5 days preoperation

   Neomycin — 2 days preoperation

5.   Explanation and reassurance to the patient

Postoperative care

1.   Rectal tube (generally removed as patient recovers, 3 - 4 days)
2.   Sedation/analgesia
3.   Much reassurance/guidance during gradual introduction of bowel function.

Complications

1.   Ascending infection (pyelonephritis)
2.   Ureteric stenosis
3.   Metabolic disturbance (general ill health, reabsorption of chemicals excreted by the kidneys e.g. chlorides).

Urinary diversion to abdominal wall

It is unusual for the ureter to be brought directly to the skin surface. It is more usual to find the ureters joined to a free piece of small bowel and this brought to the skin surfaces in the form of an ideal conduit.

Management of the patient undergoing this form of urinary diversion involves the ward team working in close harmony with the stoma care sister. She should be informed of any patient undergoing this surgery as soon as possible, as she will want to introduce herself and develop a rapport with the patient as early as she can. The sister usually asks if the spouse would like to be present during an explanatory interview.

Prior to the operation the stoma sister will mark the stoma site on the skin, so that when attached, the stoma bag does not fall into skin folds, undermining its water tight seal. Marking the skin when the patient is on the theatre table is impossible, as the skin is stretched. Two sites are usually marked to give the surgeon an alternative place to fashion the stoma.

Some stoma therapists do patch tests with adhesives to check for allergic reaction. The patient is asked if he would like to meet a person with an ileal conduit already returned to normal life.

Preoperative care

1.   Pubic and abdominal shave

2.   Bowel preparation is essential. Eash surgeon has his own preference for bowel preparation but elements involved include:

    a.   Evacuation to reduce bowel content, (enemas and high colonic washouts, e.g. castor oil, 45 ml orally, 2 days preoperation; mannitol 20 mg/250 ml in water orally (drunk in one go), about 3 days preoperation.

    b.   Reduced dietary intake. A low residue diet up to 2 days preoperation, then elemental diet, e.g. Triosorbon and tea only, up to 1 day preoperation.

    c.   Bowel sterilization, e.g. neomycin, 1 g orally, three times a day, 3 days preoperation; metronidazole (Flagyl) suppositories, 1 g 1 hour preoperation. Sometimes, retention enemas of 50% strength povidone-iodine (Betadine) are used.

    d.   Prophylactic antibiotic therapy, e.g. metronidazole (Flagyl) 200 mg orally, 3 days preoperation, followed by tobramycin 120 mg postoperation.

3.   Anti-emboli stockings are sometimes preferred by surgeons, together with anticoagulant therapy, e.g. heparin (Minihep) injections, 5000 IU three times daily.

Procedure

The patient is placed head down. A suture line is made on the opposite side to the stoma (usually paramedian). A shorter internal length and a good external spout on the conduit makes management easier. A loop of ileum is isolated with its mesentery blood supply and brought to the skin surface. Rarely, jejunum or colon is used, for example following preoperative irradiation. The ileum continuity is retained by an end-to-end anastomosis. The piece of ileum is carefully sutured to the skin surface to avoid prolapse (Fig. 18).

    An appliance is usually fitted at operation to suit the diameter of the stoma and is joined to an hourly urine monitor to record accurately the urine output, and to avoid leaks in the early phase post-surgery.

Postoperative care

This is a two fold process:

1.   General surgical management
2.   Stoma management (urinary)

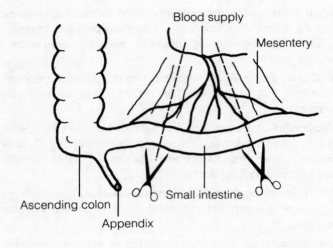

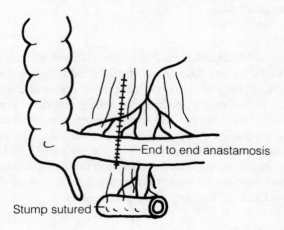

Figure 18. Formation of an ileal conduit

General surgical management. The general surgical management is similar to that for a patient undergoing major abdominal general surgery.

1. Oral intake. Nil orally initially, but gradually increasing through 30 ml/ hour to free fluids. For the patient's comfort, some surgeons allow 30 ml/ hour orally prior to nasogastric aspiration.

2. Observations. Temperature, pulse and respiration, and blood pressure are usually monitored 4-hourly following immediate postoperative phase.

3. Intravenous intake. This is normally through a subclavian or internal jugular vein. Intravenous feeding is usually required for at least 7 days.

4. Nasogastric aspiration. This is usually continued as for any postoperative bowel surgery.

5. Wound management. General observation with checks for any abdominal distention and degree of wound drainage via wound drains.

6. Oxygen therapy and physiotherapy. The patient is generally in the older age group and often initially requires regular chest physiotherapy and oxygen therapy.

7. Adequate analgesia. Usually maintained by drugs.

8. General postoperative care, including pressure area relief and mouth care.

9. Reassurance and encouragement. Teaching the patient his own stoma care, giving all the pertinent information, maintaining family involvement, informing the patient of voluntary associations (Urinary Conduit Association who offer support and will make hospital and home visits).

Stoma management (urinary) Initially hourly urine monitoring is continued but as the patient's condition improves, monitoring is reduced. Some consultants insert two ureteric splints into the urinary stoma which remain in situ 7 - 10 days.

The stoma is a permanent condition and the aim of management following the initial postoperative phase is to find the most suitable appliance for the patient and to be supportive to the patient.

Phosphatic deposits from the urine can build up on the stoma, crystallize and cut into the mucosa. If this is left untreated, the tissue will heal by fibrosis and may cause stoma stenosis. When changing the appliance dabbing the stoma with ordinary household vinegar will dissolve these deposits. A few drops of household vinegar in the urostomy bag also helps reduce any smell from stale urine.

The care of the stoma is made more difficult as urine is continually draining. Protection of the skin is important. A skin preparation protective film is most helpful. The bag seal is undermined if the surface skin around the stoma is wet when applying the bag. A useful tip is to fill a large medicine cup with tissues and apply it over the stoma. This soaks up the urine while ensuring that the skin surface is dry before the bag is applied.

The stoma often has a large mucous ooze which is removed during routine care. Mucous dispersal fluids, which can be dropped into the urinary appliance can be obtained, but these are not readily available in this country. Cloudiness of the urine is not therefore indicative of urinary tract infection.

If a specimen of urine is required for culture and sensitivity, it is useless to send a specimen from the bag, as this is often contaminated. To obtain a true specimen a narrow urethral catheter should be inserted gently into the stoma until the holes are covered and the freshly collected urine sent for analysis.

These patients usually benefit from wearing a belt to support the bag. This reduces the strain on the adhesive caused by the weight of urine in the bag.

Although the choice of bags for urostomy care is less than that available for colostomies, individual patient needs must be assessed. There is no perfect bag suitable for all users, and some bags will be better suited to some patients than others. Trial and error is the most frequent method used to find the most suitable appliance.

Different bags are designed specifically to cope with different stomas. A patient with urinary diversion cannot wear an ileostomy or colostomy bag with safety.

Urinary bags. Urinary bags have a small tube or tap outlet at the lower end of the appliance. A fairly common complaint from patients is leakage, often due to the fact that the gasket size is too big. This may be overcome by using a bag with a smaller aperture, or using a bag with a non-return valve, as it can reduce the chances of the bag leaking.

Rubber bags are sometimes used and preferred. They are used for up to 2 months and require careful washing with soapy water followed by good rinsing and drying. Unfortunately these bags need strong fingers and good eyesight to be applied and used effectively.

Some bags are made in one piece. The adhesive is an integral part of the bag e.g. Hollister bags. Others are made of two pieces where the flange and bag are separate items, e.g. Surgicare system. The choice of bag depends upon the patient's abilities and prognosis. It is no good offering a complicated system if the patient's condition is likely to make coping and independence difficult.

Problems associated with urinary diversion include:

Appliance/stoma management	*Surgical management*
Skin maceration	Wound infection
Leakage	Burst abdomen
Encrustation of stoma	Ureteric leak; peritonitis
Bleeding (minimal capillary loss	Ureteric obstruction
can be expected and is normal)	Haemorrhage
Fitting difficulties	Stoma stenosis
Hair in stoma vicinity	Acidosis
Allergy to adhesive	Intestinal obstruction
Smell	Pyelonephritis
Psychological and sexual problems, e.g.	Uretero-ileal obstruction
embarrassment, feeling of	Parastomal hernia
uncleanliness	Retraction of stoma
Acceptance of stoma	Hernia (incisional)
Supply of suitable bags	Calculi formation
	Uraemia
	Insufficient blood supply
	to stoma (loop necrosis)

Further reading

Anderson E R (1977) Women and cystitis (prevention and treatment), Nursing 7(4): 50-53

Barnett D E et al (1978) Urinary Conduit Association, Nursing Times 74 (47):1937

Breckman B (1981) Stoma care after cystectomy and ileal conduit formation (Nursing Care Study), Nursing Times 77 (26): 1110-1114

Campbell D (1982) Chronic cystitis, personal patient's experience, Nursing Mirror 155 (4): 50

Glasham R W (1982) Bladder cancer, Practitioner 226 (1373): 1891-1898

Grey A J (1980) Urinary diversion and cystectomy (Nursing Care Study), Nursing Times 76 (37): 1616-1620

Hadfield J (1981) Haematuria, clinical forum, urological emergencies, Nursing Mirror 152 (4): supplt

Hall R R (1983) Nonsurgical treatment of solid tumours, 7. Bladder cancer, Hospital Update 9 (3): 317-324

Jackson A S (1980) A conduit for life (Nursing Care Study), Nursing Times 76 (36): 1564-1567

Jones M A et al (1980) Life with an ileal conduit: results of a questionnaire, British Journal of Urology 52 (1): 21-25

Kilmartin A (1973) Understanding cystitis, Heinemann

Knowles R C Virden J E (1980) Handling of injectable antineoplastic agents, British Medical Journal 281 (6240): 589-91

Ozanne S (1982) Cystectomy: going home (Nursing Care Study), Nursing Mirror 154 (17): 56-59

Philp N H et al (1980) Ileal conduit urinary diversion, long term follow up in adults, British Journal of Urology 52 (6): 515-519

Riddle P R (1981) Urothelial tumours, Hospital Update 7 (9): 909-920

Riley A J (1983) Drugs which act on the bladder, British Journal of Sexual Medicine 10 (95): 22-28

Smith P (1978) Prostatic and bladder syndrome 2. Bladder neck obstruction, Nursing Times 74 (24): 1007-1009

Spraggon E M (1975) Urinary diversion stomas: a guide for patients and nurses, Churchill Livingstone

Wright E (1983) Double indemnity (Nursing Care Study), Nursing Mirror 156 (15): 46-49

Useful address
The Urinary Conduit Association
The Christie Hospital and Holt Radium Institute
Wilmslow Road
Manchester 20
(061-445-8123)

CHAPTER 9

KIDNEY DISEASE

The treatment of renal conditions has become very specialized. Many hospitals renal units have to care for the many patients with long-term renal problems, dialysis and transplantation.

Acute renal failure
The management of acute renal failure is very much the domain of a specialized renal unit and most surgical/urological units do not possess the necessary expensive specific equipment.

In acute renal failure the kidneys suddenly cease to produce urine in adequate quantities (oliguria) or completely (anuria). The blood urea rises rapidly, as the kidneys are actively involved with waste product excretion and electrolyte balance. Unless the balance is quickly restored, the condition can be life-threatening. Infection can prove a serious complication in these patients and the toxic effects of many drugs can make treatment difficult.

The nephron will not produce urine if:

1. The blood pressure is too low — pre-renal failure (anuria)
2. The kidney substance is damaged — renal failure (anuria)
3. There is obstruction to the urinary outflow — post-renal failure (anuria).

Causes

Pre-renal failure
1. Hypovolaemia (bleeding, vomit, diahorrea, burns
2. Cardiogenic shock (severe myocardial infarction)

3.   Bacteraemic shock (bloodborne infection)

Renal failure

1.   Nephrotoxic agents (drugs)
2.   Disseminated intravascular coagulation (septicaemia, emboli) (The clotting process and break down of clots work against one another)
3.   Incompatible blood transfusion
4.   Jaundice

Post renal failure

1.   Calculi
2.   Blood clots
3.   Tumour
4.   Prostatic enlargement
5.   Urethral obstruction

Signs and symptoms

Urine output falls (oliguria). The duration varies from hours to weeks, leading to anuria. Catheterization does not reveal urine, differentiating this condition from retention. Acute renal failure affects the body's systems, e.g. gastrointestinal (anorexia, nausea, vomiting, hiccoughs), cardiovascular (fluid and electrolyte imbalance), neuromuscular (irritability, lethargy leading to sleepiness and coma, due to uraemia), depresed immunity. Other symptoms relate to any underlying disease, e.g. rapid pulse in shock.

Treatment

The basis of treatment is to investigate and, if possible, treat the underlying cause. Specific aspects of management, to maintain life until the kidneys recover their function, are many.

Fluid balance Accurate fluid balance monitoring is vital. Urine is monitored hourly and fluid replacement is geared toward this measurement. Diuretic therapy by intravenous injection is sometimes prescribed, usually in high doses. Fluid replacement often follows a pattern of:

1. Replacing by intravenous therapy the total of one hour's urine output over the next hour.

2. Replacing approximately 500 ml extra (insensible loss). Sometimes this is given orally to maintain oral hygiene. Intravenous dextrose 20% or 50% with added soluble insulin is given for two main reasons — it boosts calorific intake, and influences electrolyte loss, by acting as a transporter encouraging the passage of calories and electrolytes across cell membranes. Potassium transport is particularly important as hyperkalaemia can lead to cardiac arrest.

    If the patient is sweating profusely, this is accounted for when calculating the total intake volume.

Electrolyte monitoring Blood samples are frequently taken to monitor urea, electrolytes and glucose levels. 24-hour urine collections for urea, electrolytes and creatine clearance are also taken.

Daily weighing The patient's weight is invaluable as a guide to fluid balance.

Drug therapy Drug therapy is used:

1. To control excessive protein breakdown e.g. nandrolone (Drabolin) up to 50 mg daily intramuscular injection. Some units use hydrocortisone injection.

2. To encourage diuresis and prevent tubular necrosis e.g. 20% mannitol infusion 200 ml or frusemide (Lasix) 250 mg intravenous injection.

3. To remove excess potassium from the body e.g. polystyrene sulphonate resin (Resonium) 15 g (a powder mixed with water) three times daily; sometimes given nasogastrically or rectally in enema form.

Diet Current dietary trends try to reduce protein intake, so if the patient is tolerating the diet a low protein meal is given. Some urologists, however, do not limit the patient's protein intake in order to maintain serum albumen levels, but this is not conventional treatment.

A low salt/potassium diet may be required and 'Hycal' type drinks are sometimes given to increase calorie intake.

The oliguric phase can continue for as long as several weeks and as the nephrons heal, urine output increases with dramatic effect. During the diuretic phase the urine is usually very dilute but concentration improves with kidney recovery.

Dialysis

If, however, the patient's condition continues to fail and the doctors need to pursue active treatment, artificial renal function (dialysis) is required.

This technique is usually performed in a renal unit or intensive care unit and employs osmotic exchange to reduce the blood poisons e.g. urea. There are two main types: haemodialysis (artificial kidney) and peritoneal dialysis.

Haemodialysis In a haemodialysis machine, layers of cellophane providing a semipermeable membrane are primed to eliminate air, and heparinized to prevent clotting of the patient's blood. The blood is transferred from the patient to the dialysis machine by a cannula and then returned to the venous system by a separate cannula. Different techniques allow for this, e.g. arteriovenous internal (subcutaneous) shunt, arteriovenous fistula and external Schribner shunt.

Circulating within the 'artificial kidney' is a dialysis fluid which attracts the metabolic end products and salts across the semipermeable membrane, from the area of higher concentration (blood) to that of lower concentration (dialysis fluid).

The composition of the dialysis fluids can be varied to control absorption/ reabsorption of electrolytes. If long-term dialysis is required, the patient usually has a "shunt" made betwen artery and vein to enable easier repeated cannulation.

Peritoneal dialysis (Fig. 19) This method of aiding renal function relies upon the permeable capacity of the patient's own peritoneum. A special peritoneal dialysis cannula is inserted through the abdominal wall just below the umbilicus and secured in place.

Dialysis fluid, e.g. Dialaflex, is warmed to body temperature in a water bath and run into the abdomen. It is left in situ to allow transfer and excretion of toxic substances to occur and then allowed to drain into a collecting bag.

Complications may include abdominal discomfort, fluid leakage, pain and peritonitis.

Patients undergoing peritoneal dialysis often require intensive nursing, but fairly recent developments allow continuous ambulatory peritoneal dialysis in suitable long-term patients. The patients are shown how to continue the treatment of connecting and using dialysis fluid bags through a permanent catheter into the abdomen.

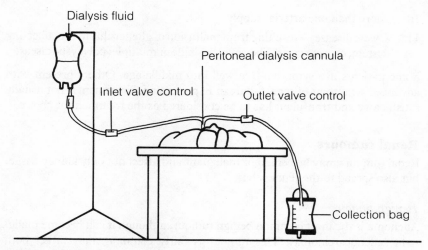

Figure 19. Diagram to show patient receiving peritoneal dialysis

Congenital kidney abnormalities

Congenital kidney abnormalities include:

1. Lack of kidneys (failure to develop) — rare, usually discovered in stillborn infants

2. Aplasia — small, not fully developed, kidneys

3. Hypoplastic kidney — not full size, but fully developed, kidney

4. Simple ectopic (pelvic) kidney — kidney not in correct position at birth, occasonally causing pain or infection

5. Fusion or horseshoe kidneys — kidneys joined together. They may cause stagnation of urine at the point of connection, with a danger of stone formation or hydronephrosis. Can be surgically separated

6. The kidneys may be fused or both lie on one side of the body

7. Malrotation — kidneys lie in the correct place but are rotated

8. Single kidney — only presents a problem if disease develops. More common than bilateral absence

9. Double ureters and/or kidneys — treatment for this is reserved if or until symptoms occur

10. More than one arterial supply
11. Cystic disease — resulting from malfusion of glomerulus to the collecting system, causing cysts. They may be single or multiple (polycystic disease).

Some patients live symptom-free well into middle-age. Others present with advanced symptoms of renal failure or hypertension. Treatment is not usually satisfactory and transplant has to be considered as the treatment of choice.

Renal tumours

Renal tumours may be benign or malignant and affect not only kidney tissue, but also spread to the renal pelvis.

Benign tumour

Adenoma is the most common benign tumour, although it can become malignant (adenocarcinoma). This tumour is fairly common, may affect both kidneys, is asymptomatic and is often found at post-mortem. It affects both men and women and its frequency increases with age.

Malignant tumour

The most common malignant growth of the kidney is adenocarcinoma (sometimes called Grawitz tumour, or hypernephroma). It tends to affect men twice as often as women, usually after 40 years of age. It may spread to the renal pelvis and tissue surrounding the kidney causing secondary deposits by spread through lymphatic and blood vessels.

Wilm's tumour is a malignant tumour affecting children.

Signs and symptoms

Signs and symptoms usually appear late and include:

1. Haematuria
2. Back ache
3. Loin swelling
4. Renal colic (from blood clot).

Investigations

1. Clinical history

2. Physical examination
3. Straight abdominal x-ray
4. Intravenous pyelogram
5. Renal arteriogram
6. Ultrasound scan
7. Bone/renal scan
8. Retrograde pyelogram
9. X-rays of spine and pelvis (to eliminate secondary deposits)

Treatment
1. Surgical removal (nephrectomy, ureterectomy). If diagnosis is confirmed by selective arteriography, some surgeons prefer the kidney to be embolized (infarcted) before surgery. A material such as a specific foam (Gelfoam) is injected under x-ray control through the renal artery to obstruct mechanically the blood supply to the kidney. It is thought that this makes the operation easier, there is less bleeding and decreasing tumour size. The gel is injected less than three days preoperatively. It carries a risk of such complications as infection and severe pain if carried out much earlier.
2. Irradiation (pre-or postoperatively as a palliative measure).

Pyelonephritis

Pyelonephritis is a common, acute bacterial infection. It affects the renal pelvis and kidney substance and may involve one or both kidneys. It may also affect the urethra, bladder and ureters. The causative organism is usually *E.coli,*

Causes
1. Urinary tract obstruction
2. Pregnancy
3. Calculi
4. Congenital abnormalities
5. Bloodborne infection

Signs and symptoms
1. Temperature elevation

2. Sweating
3. Burning on passing urine
4. Pain in the loin
5. Urgency
6. Nocturia
7. Anorexia
8. Headaches
9. Alteration in blood pressure
10. Haematuria
11. Vomiting (sometimes)
12. Rigors

Investigations

1. Initial: Midstream specimen of urine
2. When settled: Intravenous pyelogram
    Cystoscopy — retrograde pyelogram (to exclude stones)
    Blood (to assess kidney function)

Treatment

1. Bed rest
2. Fluids in large volumes
3. Antibiotics

Complications

1. Chronic pyelonephritis — renal failure
2. Abscess formation

Hydronephrosis

Hydronephrosis is a condition where the pelvis of the kidney dilates as a result of obstruction within the urinary tract. The kidney can become distended. Pyonephrosis is infected hydronephrosis.

Causes

These include any obstruction of the renal tract, e.g.:

1. Ureter — stones
   — infection (scarring)
   — tumour
2. Bladder — tumour
3. Kidney — horseshoe kidney
4. Prostate — carcinoma
   — hypertrophy
5. Urethra — stricture
   — urethral congenital obstruction.

Signs and symptoms

Signs and symptoms may present gradually as the condition develops. Hydronephrosis may remain symptom-free.

More acute problems include:

1. Back ache
2. Haematuria
3. Palpable kidney
4. Increase of fluid intake aggravating pain.

Investigations

1. Midstream specimen of urine — investigate for urinary tract infection
2. X-ray — straight abdominal, intravenous and retrograde pyelograms
3. Ultrasound of the abdomen

Treatment

1. Antibiotics if urinary tract infection present
2. Drainage by open operation and removal of the excessive portion of the renal pelvis (pyeloplasty)

Complications

1. Pyonephrosis
2. Renal failure

Renal injury

The kidneys are only small organs and although quite well protected by fat, they can be injured. Kidney injuries often result from a kick or fall on the loin. They are often damaged in road traffic accidents, although this is usually associated with multiple injury involving other organs. The more open type of injury caused by gunshot or knife wounds is less common.

Damage to the kidneys can vary in degree:

1. The kidney substance damaged but the capsule (outer covering) intact
2. The kidney substance and capsule damaged
3. The kidney substance, outer capsule and renal pelvis injured
4. Total destruction of kidney
5. Severing of the kidney from the renal artery and vein.

Signs and symptoms

1. Shock caused by blood loss
2. Pain in the back or loin
3. Swollen and tender loins
4. Bruising
5. Haematuria, varying from microscopic to very dark, dependent on the degree or damage

Investigations

X-ray — Intravenous urogram

— retrograde pyelogram

— arteriogram

Some form of diagnostic x-ray is urgently required to plan the patient's treatment.

Treatment

1. Bedrest — continuing usually for several days. Extent of haematuria governs time of mobilization
2. Pain relief — morphine often used
3. Observations — half hourly blood pressure, temperature pulse and respirations
4. Save urine samples to assess degree of haematuria. There is a risk of secondary haemorrhage
5. Haemoglobin, group and crossmatch blood
6. Regular midstream specimens of urine. If the kidneys are bruised the haematoma may get infected
7. High fluids intake — intravenous plasma or plasma expanders; whole blood if bleeding is severe. Oral fluids are not usually given initially in case a general anaesthetic is required later.

Complications

1. Persistent haematuria
2. Anaemia usually treated with iron tablets
3. High blood pressure due to degree of renal damage

The follow-up of these possible complications is usually continued as an outpatient.

Surgery Not all renal trauma patients require surgery, but some may require:

1. Repair of kidney capsule or cortex
2. Partial nephrectomy
3. Total nephrectomy.

Disease of the ureter

Disease of the ureter alone is very uncommon. Tumours are rare unless there is invasion from another site. An operation to re-implant ureters in children with urinary reflux is fairly common but in adults the most frequently seen condition is ureter injury.

Ureter injury

Ureter damage may occur at the same time as kidney injury, e.g. from penetration wounds or road traffic accidents, but it can also occur as a complication of abdominal surgery if damaged accidentally.

Signs and symptoms

Signs and symptoms relate to the kidney if there is any renal injury. If the ureter only is damaged, oliguria and renal pain may occur.

Investigations

If the ureter is damaged at the same time as the kidney, it will be revealed during the investigations for renal trauma.

If the patient is to have surgery in the pelvic area a preoperative intravenous pyelogram may be done to assess position of the ureters. A postoperative intravenous pyelogram will be performed if damage is suspected.

Treatment

Some degree of surgery may be required.

1. If stricture present — dilatation of ureter
2. If ureter damaged

    — end-to-end anastamosis

    — T-tube inserted to help relieve damage (similar to that of gall bladder surgery)

    — loop of bowel used to bridge a gap in the ureter

    — a Boari flap operation (a flap of bladder used to substitute a lower part of the ureter is implanted in the bladder).

Operations of the kidney and ureter

Nephrectomy

Nephrectomy is the removal of the kidney. The operation is usually performed through a loin incision but sometimes an abdominal incision is used.

Reasons for operation

1. Neoplasm
2. Calculi
3. Congential abnormality
4. Trauma
5. Nonfunctioning kidney (e.g. chronic infection)
6. Tuberculosis
7. Obstruction (e.g. hyronephrosis)

Preoperative care

Pre-and postoperative care encompass all the needs of a patient undergoing major surgery but specific aspects include:

1. Explanation and reassurance to patient
2. Careful monitoring and testing of urine
3. Preoperative midstream specimen of urine
4. Blood for group - and crossmatch
5. Intravenous pyelogram. This has usually been performed during patient investigation or as an emergency in traumatic cases. The films must accompany the patient to theatre.
6. Suppositories to clear bowel
7. Adequate shave including abdomen and loin
8. Antibiotic therapy if infection is suspected or present.

Postoperative care

1. Analgesia
2. Monitor wound drainage (drains usually removed within 48 hours)
3. Chest physiotherapy — discomfort can cause patient to refrain from fully expanding lungs. The patient is positioned initially on affected side to aid drainage, but is quickly transferred to semi-upright position to prevent lung complications

4. Regular dressing inspection to observe for haemorrhage

5. Patients are not usually catheterised, therefore ensure patient passes urine, observe for haematuria and obtain an- early postoperative midstream specimen of urine

6. Fluids are usually allowed freely once the patient is alert, to encourage good urine output

7. Sutures removed after 7-10 days

8. Mobilization is usually gentle, with slowly increasing activity from 36-48 hours postoperatively.

9. Normal diet

NOTE: It is vital that the patient realizes he has now only one kidney and he must carry some form of warning in case of accident (e.g. Talisman charm)

Complications

1. Haemorrhage (primary (reactionary) or secondary)

2. Paralytic ileus

3. Bowel fistula, if surgery has been difficult

4. Respiratory problems

5. Wound infection (e.g. abscess formation)

Nephro-ureterectomy

Nephro-ureterectomy is the removal of the kidney and the whole of the ureter. The pre- and postoperative care is similar to that for nephrectomy. An additional groin/suprapubic incision for the operation is made.

Reasons for operation

1. Tumour

2. Abnormal ureters

3. Calculi causing pyonephrosis

4. Tuberculosis

Preoperative care

As for nephrectomy

Postoperaive care

1. Drains. Usually one drain to kidney bed, as for nephrectomy, sometimes drain is inserted to the side of the bladder near point at which ureter has been removed. The drain is removed by shortening.
2. Patient is usually catheterized — removed after about 8 days.

Complications Damage to iliac blood vessels may occur.

Partial nephrectomy

Partial nephrectomy is the removal of part of the kidney that is diseased, leaving the healthy tissue intact.

Reasons for operation

1. Calculi
2. Trauma
3. Tuberculosis

Preoperative care As for total nephrectomy

Postoperative care

1. As for total nephrectomy.
2. Drain is usually left in a little longer and is removed by shortening from about 4 days postoperation.
3. Careful observation for urinary leak (drainage).

Complications

1. Urinary fistula
2. Heavy bleeding necessitating total nephrectomy

Nephrolithotomy

Nephrolithotomy is the removal of a stone from the body of the kidney. It is usually performed if a pyelolithomy (see p.134) is not possible.

The management of the patient closely follows that for partial nephrectomy.

Reasons for operation Calculi in the kidney substance.

Preoperative care

1. As for nephrectomy
2. Investigations (see renal calculi p.138)
3. Patient is often x-rayed en route to theatre to establish the immediate preoperative position of calculi

Postoperative care

1. As for nephrectomy
2. Drainage to kidney bed
3. Nephrectomy tube/catheter — careful observation of urinary output via tube, which can usually be discontinued after about 4 days if drainage has settled. Oedema of the tissue at the site of operation makes watertight suturing impractical.

Complications

1. Haemorrhage (reactionary or secondary)
2. Urinary fistula
3. Re-occurrence of calculi
4. Anuria

Pyelolithotomy

Pyelolithotomy is the removal of a stone through the wall of the renal pelvis.

Preoperative care As for nephrolithotomy

Postoperative care

1. As for nephrolithotomy
2. Analgesia, usually pethidine (blood, especially clots, coming down the ureter can cause colic pains)
3. The wound usually heals well

Complications Urinary fistula

Pyeloplasty

Following treatment for hydronephrosis, pyeloplasty is performed to remove excess tissue and refashion the renal pelvis.

Pre- and postoperative care

1. As for nephrolithotomy
2. A fine drainage or T-tube type drain may be used to splint the sutured ureter. This allows urine to divert into a drainage bottle, usually without suction. The tube will also allow postoperative x-rays with contrast medium to assess repair and progress. Drain removal can take more than 10 days.

Ureterolithotomy

Ureterolithotomy is the removal of a stone from the ureter

Pre- and postoperative care As for pyelolithotomy

Nephrostomy

Nephrostomy is the drainage of the kidney by, most commonly, a self-retaining catheter inserted through the renal pelvis. It is usually a temporary measure.

Reasons

1. Gross pyonephrosis
2. Postoperative care, after e.g. pyelolithotomy
3. Bilateral ureteric obstruction

Specific postinsertion care Careful urine output monitoring. Diuresis may follow the relief of obstruction.

Complications

1. Stone formation
2. Infection
3. Haemorrhage

Further reading

Ackrill P (1981) How to insert a peritoneal dialysis cannula, British Journal of Hospital Medicine 25(4): 411 413

Ainge R M (1981a) Continuous ambulatory peritoneal dialysis, Nursing Times 77 (38): 1036-1038

Ainge R M (1981b) Intermittent peritoneal dialysis, Nursing Times 77 (43): 1839-1840

Chang M (1981) Peritoneal dialysis (How patients are trained in CAPD), Nursing Mirror 153 (25): 22-25

Datta P K (1978) Hydronephrosis, Nursing Times : 1393-1395

(1982) Disabilities and how to live wth them, continuous ambulatory peritoneal dialysis, Lancet 1 (8271): 556

Durno S (1982) Left nephrectomy (Nursing Care Study), Nursing Times 78 (27): 1139-1145

Fernando O N Adams A (1976) Renal transplantation, Nursing Times 72 (41): 1598-1600

Harvey A (1979) Blunt renal trauma (Nursing Care Study of Two Patients), Nursing Times 75 (41): 1756-1758

Marwood R (1983a) Sexual problems in renal disease, Modern Medicine 28 (3): 35-36

Marwood R (1983b) Problems facing women with chronic renal failure, Modern Medicine 28 (4): 51-52

Oag D et al (1976) Chronic renal failure, Nursing Times 72 (24): 926-938

Platzer H (1980) A patient suffering from chronic renal failure, Nursing Times 76 (5): 191-195

Sanderson M (1976) Diet and dialysis, Nursing Times 72 (45): 1774-1775

Stevens E et al (1981a) 1-20 Twenty part series, Nursing Times

Stevens E (1981b) Haemodialysis I (history and development), Nursing Times 77 (22): 942-944

(1981) The symposium on renal disease, Practitioner 225 (1357): 959-1038

Teasdale C et al (1982) Arterial embolization in renal carcinoma — a useful procedure, British Journal of Urology 54 (6)' 616-619

Winder L (1980) Renal failure (Nursing Care Study), Nursing Mirror 150 (1): 37-39

(1976) X-rays in focus — post basic, Nursing Times 72 (36): supplt

(1976) X-rays in focus — post basic, Nursing Times 73 (20): supplt

CHAPTER 10

URINARY TRACT CALCULI

Calculi or stones may occur at any point within the renal tract. Urine is a very concentrated solution and can predispose to precipitation of its contents. Factors leading towards this are:

1. Increased excretion of calcium oxalate, urate and cystine (an amino acid), all of which clump either together or collect individually to form a stone e.g. calcate stone, urate stone (gout)
2. Urinary stasis, i.e. urine stagnating at some point
3. Infection — some bacteria can affect the normal urine contents
4. Kidney disease
5. Old age
6. Excess of stone-forming substances, e.g. calcium, cystine
7. Hyperparathyroidism, results in increased blood calcium

Renal calculi

Signs and symptoms

1. Colic/renal pain. Colic pain is a severe pain of sudden onset in spasms which shoot into the abdomen and groin. It can be so severe that it makes the patient curl up in a ball and often roll about in severe distress. It is often accompanied by sweating and vomiting.
2. A patient comes to the hospital with a history of passing the stone
3. Urinary tract infection
4. Haematuria

5.   Incidental x-ray finding

Investigations

1.   Clinical history, e.g. pain, renal enlargement on examination, blood pressure abnormality, rectal examination
2.   Midstream specimen of urine
3.   Blood tests including haemoglobin, full blood count, urea and electrolytes, erythrocyte sedimentation rate
4.   Stone analysis, if stone passed and collected
5.   Abdominal x-ray
6.   Intravenous urogram/pyelogram
7.   Cystoscopy, and sometimes retrograde pyelogram
8.   24-hour collection of urine for measurement of calcates, urates and phosphates

Treatment

Treatment can depend upon a number of factors:
1.   Size. A tiny stone may not require immediate treatment but one increasing in size does
2.   Pain and haemorrhage
3.   Recurrent infection
4.   Obstruction, most commonly at the exit of the pyramid or renal pelvis
5.   Age
6.   Degree of kidney damage.

If the stone does not warrant immediate surgery, regular x-rays and clinic appointments are arranged to monitor its development.

Conservative treatment

1.   Analgesia — commonly pethidine injection
2.   Abundant fluids — 2.5-3 litres daily to 'flush' out the stone
3.   Urine filtration — if the stone is passed it can be analysed
4.   Low calcium diet — if indicated by high urinary calcium levels

5. Low oxalate diet — i.e. no spinach, strawberries, chocolate or rhubarb if indicated by high urinary oxalate levels

Surgical Treatment

1. Nephrectomy — removal of kidney
2. Nephro-ureterectomy — removal of kidney and whole ureter — uncommon
3. Partial nephrectomy — removal of part of kidney

4. Nephrolithotomy — removal of stone from kidney
5. Pyelolithotomy — removal of stone through the wall of the renal pelvis — more common

Stones in the ureter

Stones in the ureter are less common than kidney stones, but may sometimes become impacted in the ureter. Some stones with jagged edges can impact to form 'stag horn' calculi which require surgical removal. They are renal in origin.

Signs and symptoms

1. Pain
2. Nausea and vomiting
3. Sweating
4. Dysuria

Investigations

1. As for renal calculi
2. Retrograde pyelogram can flush out small stones if the catheter can be distal to the stone

Treatment

1. Conservative treatment — as for renal calculi
2. Surgical treatment — endoscopic removal or open surgery

Endoscopic removal Dormia basket (Fig. 20) can be employed to remove a ureteric stone that is fairly low down the ureter. A cystoscope is passed and the ureter is found. A lead with a retractable basket is then pushed down the cystoscope and up the ureter. This catches the stone, which can then be withdrawn.

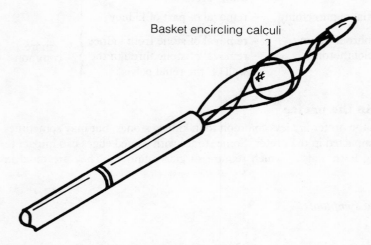

Basket encircling calculi

Figure 20. Diagram of a Dormia basket

Open surgery Open removal may be required, dependent upon

1. Stone size
2. Renal function
3. Infection
4. A non-moving stone high up the ureter

If pain and pyrexia persist, an urgent intravenous urogram is performed, and the stone has to be removed. The surgical procedures used to remove a stone include uterolithotomy. Surgery is always required if a stone perforates the ureter (indicated by extravasation of urine or an intravenous urogram/ pyelogram).

Recent work in this field has included the removal of a stone by percutaneous nephrolithotomy. Under local anaesthetic, a tract through the loin is formed and enlarged with the use of dilators to enable the passage of a nephroscope into the renal pelvis. Under direct vision the calculi is grasped and removed.

An advancement of this treatment has been the correction of pelvi-ureteric junction obstruction.

Stones can be destroyed by ultrasonic fulguration, but this use of controlled ultrasonic sound waves is still in its formative stages.

Another method suggested has been to milk stones in the lower ureter into the bladder and through the vagina in poor surgical risk female patients.

Stones in the bladder

Stones in the bladder may be single or multiple. They originate from the kidney, or have formed in the bladder due to infection in the bladder or to stasis of urine caused by

1. Prostate enlargement preventing complete outflow

2. Bladder neck obstruction

3. Foreign body (e.g. a piece of catheter can cause substances to precipitate)

4. Diverticulum in the bladder — urine can stagnate in the pouch

Signs and symptoms

1. None — stone discovered on x-ray

2. Pain — the patient usually describes some problem with micturition

3. Haematuria

4. Oliguria leading to frequency

5. Chronic cystitis caused by the stone irritating the bladder wall

Investigations

1. Physical examination

2. X-ray

3. Cystoscopy

Treatment

Treatment may be by passing a lithortrite which has jaws at the end which are used to grasp the stone and crush it. If the stone is small enough it can be flushed out with a cystoscope (Fig. 21).

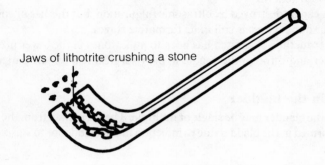

Jaws of lithotrite crushing a stone

Figure 21. Jaws of lithotrite crushing stone

Open surgery is required if:

1. The urethra is too small to pass the large lithotrite i.e. in children, or patients with urethral stricture
2. Acute cystitis is present
3. The stone is in a diverticulum
4. The stone is too large or too hard
5. Bladder tumour is present

Urethral calculi

Urethral calculi are very rare and if they do lodge, a bougie may be passed to push the stone back into the bladder. An incision can then be made to relieve it. Prostatic stones are not unknown and these can escape into the urethra.

Further reading

Bishop M C (1982a) Surgical aspects of stone disease — 1, Hospital Update 8 (4): 503-509

Bishop M C (1982b) Surgical aspects of stone disease — 2, Hospital Update 8 (5): 631-637

Hadfield J (1981) Griping about renal colic, Clinical Forum, Urological Emergencies, Nursing Mirror 152 (4): supplt

Hodgkinson A (1976) The changing pattern of urinary tract stone disease, Nursing Mirror 142 (7): 65-66

Marshall V R Ryall R L (1981) Investigation of urinary calculi, British Journal of Hospital Medicine 26 (4): 389-392

Rao P N et al (1982) Dietary management of urinary risk factors in renal stone formers, British Journal of Urology 54 (6): 578-583

Wickham J E A Kellett M J (1981) Percutaneous nephrolithotomy, British Journal of Urology 53 (4): 297-299

CHAPTER 11

URINARY TRACT INFECTION

Urinary tract infection is one of the most common infections seen in hospital. The risk of infection is much greater following catheterization (see also cystitis, p.92 and pyelonephritis, p.125)

Signs and symptoms

1. Bacteriuria
2. Frequency/nocturia
3. Dysuria/stranguary
4. Pain
5. Proteinaemia
6. 'Smelly' urine
7. Haematuria
8. Generally 'unwell'
9. Malaise
10. Headache
11. Nausea/vomiting
12. Bacteraemia
13. Rigor
14. Fever
15. Septicaemia

It should be remembered that although patients often present with a combination of these symptoms, it is a minority in whom the disease progresses to the advanced stage of bacteraemia and septicaemia.

A 'fishy' smell is often indicative of infected urine. The pain the patient feels when urinating is often described as like 'passing broken glass' or 'razor blades'. When infection reacts with the bladder wall, pus appears in the urine. If the condition ascends, pain may be felt in the perineum, suprapubic or loin region as it progresses.

Causes

Infection is much more common in women than men, because of the close proximity of the vagina and anus, which is contaminated with micro-organisms, and the shorter urethra.

Other circumstances predisposing to urinary tract infection include diabetes, pregnancy, calculi, abnormal anatomy, haematuria, instrumentation, previous urinary tract infection, previous urological surgery, family history and known renal disease.

If the patient complains of any of the above symptoms, ward testing and specimens of urine for laboratory investigations are performed immediately. Early treatment (the administration of the drug to which the causative organism is most sensitive) prevents the condition progressing to a more severe state.

Treatment

1. Co-trimoxazole (Septrin or Bactrim) 480 mg tablets, two tablets 8-12 hourly. Co-trimoxazole is a synthetic antibacterial drug which interferes with growth of bacteria. Side effects are minor gastric upset.

2. Nitrofurantoin (Furadantin) 50 mg tablets, 100 mg four times daily. Nitrofurantoin is used in the treatment of bacterial infections and should be given at or following mealtimes. It can cause nausea and vomiting and is rarely given in a course lasting over 2 weeks.

3. Nalidixic acid (Negram) 500 mg tablets, two tablets 6-hourly for 7 days, then one tablet 6 hourly. This drug is antibacterial and is used in both acute and chronic urinary infections. The commonest infecting organism, *E.coli*, is usually sensitive to this drug. Its side effects are mild but can include gastrointestinal upset.

4. Trimethoprim (Ipral) 100 mg tablets, two tablets 12-hourly or three tablets daily. This drug has similar action to co-trimoxazole.

5. Potassium citrate, 1-4 g is sometimes prescribed, though less often than formerly. It reduces the symptoms of cystitis, by reducing the acidity of the urine and therefore the burning sensation. It does not, however, arrest the infection. If any renal impairment is present it is not given, to avoid elevation in body potassium levels. Potassium citrate has also been used to replace potassium in diuretic therapy.

6. The patient should be encouraged to plenty of fluids, to flush out the bacteria.

Bacteriology

The most common organism in urinary tract infection is *Escherichia coli*, usually a harmless inhabitant of the bowel. It is not sensitive to penicillin.

White blood cells are usually present in infected urine and the white cell count is important in the detection of sterile pyuria (pus in urine) in tuberculosis investigation.

Streptococcus faecalis, a bowel bacterium, is a fairly frequently found cause of urine tract infection.

Unfortunately more resistant strains of bacteria can also cause urine tract infection including *Proteus, Pseudomonas,* and *Klebsiella* species. These tend to affect catheterized patients in a hospital environment. These species are very troublesome, resistant to many antibiotics and it is therefore essential that these bacteria are not passed on by cross-infection.

Further reading

Asscher A W (1977) Disease of the urinary system: urinary tract infection, British Medical Journal 1 (6072): 1332-1335

Casewell M (1979) Urinary tract infection, bacteria, danger on the ward, Nursing Mirror 148 (20): 37-39

Hadfield J (1980) Urological emergencies, urinary tract infection, Clinical Forum, Nursing Mirror 152 (4): supplt

Jameson R M (1976) Recurrent urinary tract infection in women, Nursing Mirror 143 (4): 55-57

Meers P D Strange J L (1980) Hospitals should do the sick no harm, No.7, Nursing Times 151 (4): supplt

Riley A J (1983a) Drugs used in the treatment of urinary tract infection - 1, British Journal of Sexual Medicine 10 (93): 16, 18

Riley A J (1983b) Drugs used in the treatment of urinary tract infection - 2, British Journal of Sexual Medicine 10 (94): 28-34

CHAPTER 12

INFERTILITY

Problems in conception will be experienced by approximately 12 couples in every 100. Sometimes the strain on the relationship this problem causes means that couples separate before consulting a doctor. Old wives' tales may be offered by friends and relatives as advice, e.g. pointing the feet towards some local landmark. To be a 'barren' woman was once a social stigma, and there is still much social pressure for married couples to have children. The causes of failure to conceive may lie with the wife, husband, or be unknown, and no one is more likely than the other.

Investigation

The present procedure to investigate infertility is for the wife to be referred to a gynaecologist, and the husband to a urologist or for one specialist to investigate the couple's problem. A detailed questionnaire is given in the initial interview, which is handled with tact to prevent distress. The aim of the initial interview is to establish that the couple's sexual activity is compatible with pregnancy. Questions are directed at both partners in order to establish the following:

1. Length of marriage (usually two years are left to elapse without using contraceptives, before investigations commence).

2. Frequency of sexual intercourse

3. Any history of pregnancy/miscarriage in the present or any previous marriage/any termination of pregnancy

4. If any type of contraception has been used, and for how long

5. If either partner has been exposed to irradiation

6. Any psychosexual disorders, e.g. loss of libido or failure to achieve

orgasm. These patients are normally referred to a specialist for counselling. Orgasm is not essential for conception in the woman

7. If there is any alcohol-related problem e.g. loss of libido

Questions specific to the woman

1. Age (fertility naturally declines with age)
2. Menstrual history (commencement of cycle, dysmenorrhoea)
3. Medical history
4. Coital difficulties, e.g. painful coitus
5. Previous surgery

Questions specific to the man

1. Medical history
2. Previous surgery
3. Difficulty with erection, penetration or ejaculation
4. Type of underwear worn (it is thought that underwear may increase heat and reduce sperm motility

Possible causes of infertility

The woman

1. Absence or abnormality of reproductive tract
2. Undiagnosed
3. Coital difficulties — any condition leading to painful coitus (dyspareunia) e.g. vaginitis, painful scars, etc.
4. Chronic infection, e.g. gonorrhoea, tuberculosis
5. Endometriosis (uterine mucosa in abnormal position in the ovary)
6. Sperm/cervical mucus incompatibility:
    a. cervical mucus very thick or scanty
    b. antibodies against sperm
7. Abnormal hormone levels disturbing menstruation/ovulation
8. Inflammatory condition blocking fallopian tubes
9. Complications of previous surgery

The man

1. Absence or abnormality of the reproductive tract
2. Undiagnosed
3. Endrocrine disorders e.g. Addison's disease
4. Varicocele — heat increased, motility of sperm decreased
5. Hydrocele — heat increased, motility of sperm decreased
6. Spermatocele — blockage of vas deferens
7. Hernia — heat increased, motility of sperm decreased
8. Undescended testes, abnormal testicle
9. Previous torsion of testes — blockage of vas
10. Phimosis — ejaculation impaired
11. Hypospadias and epispadia — ejaculation affected
12. Peyronie's disease — painful erection, difficult intercourse
13. Venereal disease — stricture formation
14. Complications of previous surgery, e.g. surgery around the bladder neck may result in retrograde ejaculation or damage to nerve supply in abdominal surgery
15. Neurological conditions

Clinical investigations

The woman

1. Physical examination
2. Tubal insufflation to determine if tubes are patent, largely superseded by laparoscopy/dye test with dilute methylene blue solution
3. Test for ovulation

    a. Endomentrium biopsy

    b. Blood hormone level estimation (follicle stimulating hormone and luteinizing hormone)

    c. Daily morning temperature (basal body temperature). Temperature rises in mid cycle, indicative of ovulation occurring

    d. Examination of cervical mucus

    e. Vaginal smear

4. Hysterosalpingography — x-ray outlining reproductive tract using contrast medium

5. Laparoscopy

The man

1. Physical examination allows the doctor to eliminate many of the listed causes, some of which could be corrected surgically. It will also highlight any features characteristic of hormone or chromosome abnormality, e.g. Cushing's syndrome.

2. Per rectum examination to investigate possible prostate or seminal vesicle disorder.

3. Semen analysis is an obligatory test, done for five main reasons:
   a. Volume — usually 2-5 ml. Reduced volume may indicate, e.g. seminal vesicle damage caused by diabetes

   b. Sperm count — usually about 60-200 million/ml. Less than 10 million makes conception almost impossible; about 20 million makes conception unlikely

   c. Appearance — usually minimal abnormality; check on the state of sperm for normality

   d. Motility — usually very active for a long time; if motility is reduced, so are chances of conception. Heat will decrease motility.

   e. Fructose — normally present in seminal vesicles and a low concentration can indicate disease at this level. This test is carried out on a fresh specimen with 2 hours of masturbation, collected in a plastic container. A rubber sheath is not used because it may sometimes contain a spermicidal lubricant and can affect sperm. Sometimes a specimen of cervical mucus is taken following intercourse to observe the motility of the sperm and eliminate sperm/mucus incompatibility. If the man is unwilling to masturbate for religious/psychological reasons, a postcoital specimen may be obtained from the vagina within 2 hours of intercourse.

4. Testicular biopsy. Patients are normally admitted to hospital for this investigation as a general anaesthetic is required. There is no special pre-operative preparation. Chromic (dissolving) stitches are usually inserted to skin as these sutures avoid the difficult removal of tiny sutures or clips.

A scrotal support is used as a routine for comfort and to help prevent scrotal haematoma. Analgesia and an anti-emetic drug e.g. prochlorperazine (Stemetil) or metoclopramide (Maxalon) are often required as this procedure produces pain often with a sickening character. The biopsy also affords full examination of the testes, epididymis and cord. Soft testes are often infertile. If there is any congenital change or absence of any part, there is no treatment. The biopsy specimen is examined under a microscope.

5.   Vasogram is an x-ray procedure, using a contrast medium to outline the vas deferens and check potency.

6.   Midstream specimen of urine tested for any chronic infection which may affect fertility

Treatment of infertility

1.   If any part of the reproductive tract is absent, there is no treatment.

2.   Surgical correction for any condition amenable to surgery e.g. correct varicocele, hernia, etc.

3.   Normal sperm production on biopsy. Often there is absence or blockage of vas or epididymis. If there is a blockage, an attempt is made to bridge the gap. Epididymovasostomy, joining the vas deferens to the epididymis, is performed if the blockage is in the vas deferens. Epididymo-epididymostomy, excising a piece of epididymis, produces results that are not optimistic. Pre- and postoperative care is as for testicular biopsy.

4.   Low sperm count. Hormone therapy sometimes helps by improving motility and count, e.g. mesterolone (ProViron). Artificial insemination may help these patients

5.   No sperm produced by testes. Nothing can be done to help these patients. Artificial insemination donor (AID) (not readily available in the National Health Service) or adoption may be discussed.

6.   Cold scrotal douches twice daily for at least 3 months. It takes 3 months for a sperm to become fully mature so treatment must be prolonged.

Further reading

Egerton P M (1976) Subfertility. Its causes and treatment. Investigations of unattained pregnancy, Nursing Times 74 (26): 1096-1099

Garrey M M et al (1978) Gynaecology Illustrated, second edition, Churchill Livingstone

Hargreave T B (1983) Male Infertility, Springer

Haslam M T (1982) Psychosexual dysfunction, Practitioner 226 (1373): 1880-1886

Khan S Ali (1983) Haematospermia, British Journal of Sexual Mediine 10 (6): 15-20

Philip E (1981) The investigation of male and female infertility, Midwife, Health Visitor and District Nurse: 12-13

Roberts A (1978) Seminal fluid and hydrocele (includes investigation for infertility), Nursing Times 74 (7): supplt

CHAPTER 13

INCONTINENCE OF URINE

This is the involuntary passing of urine in a socially undesirable place. A patient with voluntary control is not incontinent. Incontinence can sometimes be cured, but if not, it can always be made more easily manageable and improved. Much research is being conducted at present and the employment of incontinence specialist sisters helps but their workload is usually higher than he/she can manage alone.

Causes

Before treatment is considered, the true nature and pattern of the disease for each individual is required, and it is the nurse's accurate nursing assessment which highlights this. Factors contributing towards incontinence include:

1. Bladder neck weakness — often as a result of childbirth, the increased abdominal pressure caused by coughing, laughing and sneezing etc., can cause urine to escape. This is stress incontinence and it may be improved with physiotherapy.

2. Any condition leading to urgency — including pregnancy, enlarged prostate, inflamed bladder, increased fluid intake and diuretics. The bladder cannot retain urine very long before releasing it.

3. A depression of nervous control — spinal cord disease or damage. Drugs, e.g. night sedation, will reduce bladder sensation

4. Inability to reach toilet before urination is unavoidable — e.g. in severe arthritis. Treatment is to ensure that toilet facilities are within easy reach or readily available, e.g. urinal.

When investigating a patient complaining of incontinence, it is beneficial to know:

1. How much sensation the patient feels before voiding. Is there urgent desire, no desire, etc.
2. How long the patient can contain the urine before voiding occurs
3. Can the patient get to toilet facilities in time (often patients know where every public toilet is in the town so as to avoid these problems when out)
4. How effective is the bladder neck outlet (this is particularly important in stress incontinence)
5. How much control does the patient have over the bladder muscle, e.g. in cases of nerve damage.

Management
In many cases, incontinence brings with it feelings of guilt and treatment should therefore maintain the patient's dignity.

Bowels
Avoid constipation, as a full bowel can affect the urinary tract by decreasing the bladder capacity and interfere with urine outflow.

Odour
Odour occurs if urine is stale and/or concentrated. Management is aimed at preventing these problems by encouraging normal daily fluid intake and preventing urine stasis by prompt nursing aid.

Deodorant sprays are helpful and one or two deodorant drops from the single drop type onto clothing helps dispel odour, but care must be taken to avoid skin contamination.

Drinking
It is advisable for the patient to continue normal fluid intake during the daytime but use a little restraint in the evening. This will help prevent any dehydration and diminish the chance of stone formation with concentrated urine.

Skin care
Urine should be quickly washed off the skin with soap and water as it causes

soreness and redness. Harsh rubbing is best avoided. If the skin becomes cracked or dry, skin cream can be used.

Physiotherapy

Physiotherapy is useful to improve incontinence and to help retrain the bladder following catheter removal. It helps by encouraging the function of the muscles of the pelvis involved in urine control.

Pelvic floor exercises

1. Exercise 1. The patient is lying, knees bent, with his feet on the bed. He tightens the stomach and seat muscles, pulls in hard and then relaxes.
    Progressions of this exercise include tightening the stomach and seat muscles, pressing the thighs together, pulling in hard and then relaxing; tightening the stomach muscles and stretching alternate legs straight into the air; tightening the stomach muscles then stretching both legs and lowering both legs onto the bed, keeping them straight.
2. Exercise 2. The patient sits on a chair, leaning forward, hands lying between the knees. He tries to push the knees together, tightens the seat muscles, pushes the hips forward and then relaxes.
3. Exercise 3. The patient is lying down and puts one leg on top of the other. He presses top leg onto the bottom leg, tightening the muscles hard. He tightens seat and stomach muscles, then relaxes them.

These exercises aimed at stimulating the pelvic floor muscles (mainly levator ani muscle) need to be done for 15 minutes twice a day to be effective. Exercise 1 can also be done standing or walking and done as many times as possible during each day. The progressions and more strenuous exercises obviously need selection for each person's capabilities.

Encouraging the patient to stop the flow in the middle of passing urine and then restarting at each voiding after catheter removal can help with improving incontinence. The patient should also be encouraged to wait as long as possible when the desire to urinate occurs, and to try to extend the period from one urination to the next.

These exercises do take time to help but with time can afford much improvement.

Bladder drill

Bladder drill encourages the patient to pass urine at regular intervals before the urge to urinate. It is linked to each patient's individual need, e.g. hourly bladder emptying initially, progressively increased as the bladder capacity improves (Fig. 22). Fig. 23 shows a time and amount chart to show the effectiveness of bladder drill.

Instructions to Patients on Bladder Drill

You are required to:

1. Buy a notebook and a 500 ml plastic measuring jug.

2. Keep a record in the notebook of the exact time of every occasion you pass urine.

3. By passing urine into the jug, measure the volume of each amount of urine passed while at home, and if possible all the time. Record the volume against the time in the notebook.

4. To begin with, pass urine once every hour according to the time by the clock. Try to hold your water for the full hour even if you feel the need to go sooner.

5. Reduce the amount you drink in the evening and drink no further fluid after 8 pm.

6. Keep a record of every time you are incontinent whether by day or at night and record it in your notebook as either . . . damp . . . wet . . . clothes soaking.

7. If you manage to stay dry on one hourly voiding, gradually increase the time interval between passing urine from 1 hour to 1½ hours to 2 hours to 2½ hours. However always void according to the time by the clock.

This instruction leaflet is given to patients following bladder drill at home.

Figure 22. Instructions on bladder drill to patient

TIME AND AMOUNT CHART
NAME

DATE			DATE			DATE		
TIME	AMOUNT	STATE	TIME	AMOUNT	STATE	TIME	AMOUNT	STATE
TOTAL			TOTAL			TOTAL		
RESIDUAL			RESIDUAL			RESIDUAL		

Figure 23. Time and amount chart to show effectiveness of bladder drill. State refers to degree of incontinence

Appliances used in urinary incontinence

Bed pads

Disposable pads are used to treat many patients. They are cheap and readily available, and tend to be more suitable for patients who are infrequently incontinent in small amounts. The pad layers are bonded down two sides and it is important that these are placed across the bed so that fluid moves away from the patient. One of their disadvantages is that to work well there should be no clothing between pad and patient. They are, therefore, unsuitable for use out of bed because the patient is left naked below the waist.

Bed sheet

A more expensive, but much longer lasting, type of appliance is the incontinence (Kylie) bed sheet. Designed to be more comfortable by being more absorbant and preventing pooling of urine. The sheet has two distinct layers, a water repellent top layer and a highly absorbant lower layer. They need less frequent changing, lasting many hours. Their disadvantage is that they are unsuitable for patients who are doubly incontinent, and they need careful laundering.

Padding

As an additional aid to bed pads, a smaller pad often secured with elasticated briefs (Molnycke) helps management. They are useful in doubly incontinent patients.

Pants

Absorbant pants may be disposable or re-usable and allow more freedom of movement. They need to be well fitting around the waist and around the legs. They can look at times like baby pants but some do look more cosmetically pleasing. Their disadvantage is that they are fairly costly, and need regular change and attention to prevent skin problems.

For men with dribbling incontinence, a pouch (Nupron) resembling a sport supporter, is available. The waterproof pouch holds a plastic bag fitted over the penis and fastened with a velcro fastner to prevent back flow.

Pants with disposable liners (Fig. 24)

The more modern type of appliance has a pouch stitched to the outside of a tight-fitting pair of pants (Kanga), into which a disposable pad is placed. A one-

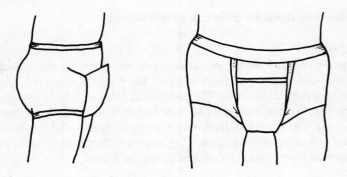

Figure 24. Pants with disposable liner (Kanga type)

way fabric prevents the patient getting wet from the pad. The pad again needs to be regularly changed and the garment needs to be close fitting to be fully effective. Their cosmetic appearance tends to lend their use more to female patients but they are not ideally suited to bedfast patients.

Collecting devices

Catheters are collecting devices but no external collecting devices are available for female patients. For male patients, a less used method is Paul's tubing. A simple length of tubing is placed over the penis and urine empties into a collecting bag.

More popular are the condom type, available on prescription, made of soft latex of different sizes to avoid leakage (Fig. 25). Their use is enhanced by the use of some type of adhesive (Conveen Uriliner). They are useless if the wrong size or incorrectly fitted. Many companies produce this type of appliance (Seton, Conveen) and ideally they need changing daily.

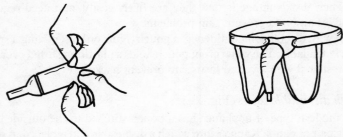

Figure 25. Condom type appliance   **Figure 26.** Rigid style collection unit (Downs)

More male collecting devices are available, made of more lasting rubber material. These require care in washing and careful fitting and therefore require a fairly high level of self care (Fig. 26)

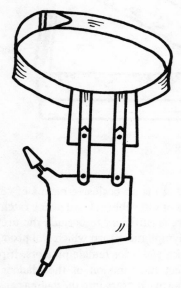

Figure 27. Collection bag suspended from waist

Catheters

Catheters tend to be used less frequently in the management of incontinence. Occasions when they may be used include: patients with some outflow obstruction (e.g. prostatic disease) who are unfit for surgery, or when all other measures are ineffective.

For drainage, a closed system is employed. The collecting bag is either strapped to the leg or supported from a belt around the waist (Wallace Holster, Barclay, Seton). These bags hang discretely beneath ordinary clothes. Their smaller capacity demands regular emptying. The importance of community management cannot be overstated. Some urologists prefer regular bladder washouts with antiseptic solution upward of twice weekly (Fig. 27).

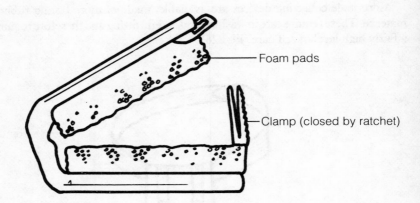

Figure 28. Penile clamp

Penile clamp

A penile clamp (Fig. 28) is an occlusive means of controlling incontinence, composed of two jaws of soft rubber closed over a ratchet. Placed at the base of the glans the pressure is sufficient to occlude the urethra yet not enough to prevent venous and lymphatic return which will produce gross swelling.

No occlusive device exists for female patients. If prolapse of the uterus is present, it may affect the function of the bladder or urethra and cause incontinence. A supportive pessary into the vagina can help restore continence.

Drugs

If the incontinence is due to urinary tract infection, the antibiotic drug to which the causative organism is sensitive is given to alleviate the problem.

If the bladder lacks tone, the resultant full bladder can produce an overflow of urine. Drug therapy is used to try and increase bladder tone.

1. Carbachol, 2 mg tablets, 1-4 mg daily
2. Bethanechol chloride (Myotinine), 5 mg, 10 mg, 25 mg tablets, 5-30 mg upto 4 times daily
3. Distigmine bromide (Ubretid), 5 mg tablets, 5 mg daily; 500 µg injection, 5 µg daily
4. Flurbiprofen (Froben), 50 mg tablets, 50 mg three times daily

If the incontinence is due to irritability of the bladder caused by small amounts of urine, it may be helped by relaxing the bladder muscle. Drugs producing this effect are:

1. Flavoxate hydrochloride (Urispas), 100 mg tablets, 200 mg three times daily
2. Emepronium bromide (Cetiprin), 100 mg, 200 mg tablets, 200 mg three times daily

Enuresis is sometimes treated by the use of imipramine (Tofranil) 25 mg tablets, 25 mg at night. Its exact effect is not fully understood. Suggestions have been that it decreases bladder excitability, and increases bladder capacity. Research is still in progress.

Electronic aids

Electronic aids are aimed at increasing muscle tone by stimulation using an electronic impulse. Intermittent electronic stimulation (faradism) may be performed rectally or vaginally. If continuous stimulation is required, permanent implants around the bladder neck may be inserted.

Surgical treatment

There are various methods of surgical treatment employed to try and achieve continence.

A prosthesis is inserted to compress the urethra. This is most commonly used in cases where there is some sphincter damage resulting from surgery or trauma. A balloon is inserted into the perineal area to push against the urethra. The patient passes urine by overcoming the resistance with muscle contraction. Its effect can be enhanced with the addition of silicone fluid.

Some prostheses are designed to control the inflation and deflation of the balloon compressing the urethra, with an additional silicone bladder with a control valve inserted into the perineal or suprapubic region. By squeezing the silicone bladder, the urethral balloon or cuff can be controlled e.g. Rosens and Brantley Scott prostheses.

No specific preoperative preparation is necessary, except a pubic shave. Thorough genital/perineal cleansing is essential. Postoperatively, the urethral catheter is left in situ for 7 - 10 days until healing is advanced.

Prosthesis function is introduced gradually. During the early postoperative phase the prosthesis cuff is left deflated to prevent necrosis of the urethral wall against the catheter.

Complications

1. Infection, which results in painful rejection of the prosthesis. This cannot be treated with antibiotics as they tend not to be effective when foreign bodies are present.
2. Cuff or mechanical failure.

A less used surgical method of compressing the urethra is to make a sling of fascia or muscle which is passing under the urethra and tightened to compress it.

Female stress incontinence can be treated surgicially, dependent upon its degree.

Operations designed to support the bladder neck because the normal muscle support is weak e.g. Marshall Marchetti, Krantz and Tonagho procedures, are more common. Preoperatively cystoscopy is performed to ensure there is no residual urine, cystitis, etc., before surgery is performed. Preoperative vulval cleansing is essential.

The correct alignment for the urethra and bladder exit is achieved by suturing vaginal tissue and pulling this upwards to given support and anchoring it with sutures to pubic periosteum or ligament. Urethral catheterization is followed by bladder drill postoperatively. General wound toilet should be performed.

Further reading

Clay E C (1978a) Incontinence I — effects of incontinence on adults, Nursing Mirror 146 (9): 14-16

Clay E C (1978b) Incontinence 2 — habit retraining, Nursing Mirror 146 (10): 36-38

Clay E C (1978c) Incontinence 3 — regime for retaining, Nursing Mirror 146 (11): 23-24

Clay E C (1978d) Incontinence 4 — management with protective clothing, Nursing Mirror 146 (12): 23-35

(1977) Incontinence. Nursing in the community, Nursing Mirror 144: supplt

(1983a) Incontinence 1, Physiotherapy 69 (4): 104-113

(1983b) Incontinence 2, Physiotherapy 69 (5): 144-149

Mandelstam D A (1977) Incontinence, Heinemann

Mandelstam D A (1979) Incontinence: the mop and bucket approach is dead, Geriatric Medicine 9 (4): 30-34

Perston Y (1981) Urinary incontinence — ways to help solve a sensitive problem, Nursing Mirror 153 (17): 38-42

Reed E A (1976) The problem of incontinence, Nursing Mirror 142 (17): 616-618

Slack P (1981) Incontinence — a forward look, Nursing Times : supplt

Willington F L (1975) Incontinence, MacMillan journals

Worth P H L (1979) Incontinence in the male patient, Practitioner 223 (1335): 325-330

Useful address

Disabled Living Foundation
346 Kensington High Street
London
W14 8N

CHAPTER 14

TUBERCULOSIS

Tuberculosis is now uncommon, usually presenting in the kidney or epididymis within the genitourinary tract. More commonly seen in the young adult, it is usually a secondary infection to a primary infection of the lung.

Kidney
The infection usually lodges in the kidney substance and forms large cavities in the kidney body. If the cavities are open-ended tubercles, the infection can spread to the rest of the genitourinary tract:

1. Ureter, which generally develops an ulcerated appearance and can become contracted
2. Bladder, which may also take on an ulcerated appearance and become contracted.

Epididymis
The epididymis can also become infected from a lung condition and may develop a hydrocele. If untreated, it can lead to the formation of a sinus.

Signs and symptoms

Upper tract
1. Backache
2. Loss of weight

3. Night sweating
4. Colic
5. Nocturia

Lower tract

1. Frequency
2. Haematuria
3. Dysuria
4. Pyrexia
5. Nocturia

Genitalia

1. Hydrocele
2. Loin pain
3. Swelling
4. Orchitis
5. Impotence
6. Infertility
7. Sinus

Investigations

1. Clinical history
2. Social history (family history, possible contact)
3. Physical examination including chest
4. Chest x-ray, abdominal/loin x-ray, intravenous pyelogram
5. Blood tests — haemoglobin, red blood cells, white cell count, erythrocyte sedimentation rate (elevated)
6. Midstream specimen and three early morning specimens of urine, usually the total volume of the first voiding of the day
7. Cystoscopy

Treatment

Surgery

1. Removal of the kidney (nephrectomy)
2. Nephrectomy and removal (nephro-ureterectomy) of full ureter
3. Removal of part of the kidney (partial nephrectomy)
4. Cavernotomy (drainage and surgical toilet to the cavities caused by the disease)
5. Bouginage of ureteric stricture (dilation of the ureter)
6. Operative excision of stricture (if bougies fail)
7. Caecocystoplasty (rarely performed operation in which a piece of caecum is used to enlarge the bladder)
8. Urinary diversion (diversion of the ureters from the bladder to sigmoid colon)

Surgery is usually delayed until the patient has had at least 2 full months of medical therapy.

Medical therapy

1. Drugs: usually required for 9-12 months to achieve 6 months clear urine. Initial treatment starts daily with rifampicin, 450-600 mg daily, orally; isoniazid, 300 mg daily, orally; para-amino-salicyclic acid (PAS) 12-15 mg daily, orally, or ethambutol 15 mg/kg daily, orally (not used in older people). Side effects include nausea, fever, giddyness, diahorrea and (uncommon) vomiting.
2. Bedrest: slowly increase exercize as temperature decreases
3. Diet

Follow-up
The doctor usually continues to see the patient over a 5-year period, although after 2-3 years, a relapse is uncommon.

Further reading

Gow J G (1979) Genitourinary tuberculosis: a 7-year review, British Journal of Urology 51 (3): 239-244

Further reading

Books

Blandy J P (1978) Transurethral resection, second edition, Pitman Medical

Blandy J P (1982) Lecture notes on urology, third edition, Blackwell Scientific

Booth J A (1983) Handbook of investigations, Harper and Row

Brunner L S Suddarth D S (1980) Textbook of medical—surgical nursing, fourth edition, Harper and Row

Goldman M (1978) A guide to the X-ray department, Wright

Gow J G Hopkins H H (1978) Handbook of urological endoscopy, Churchill Livingstone

Lloyd-Davies R W Gow J G Davies D R (1983) A colour atlas of urology, Wolfe

McConnell E A Zimmerman M F (1983) Care of patients with urological problems, Lippincott

Scott R Deane R Callander R (1982) Urology illustrated, second edition, Churchill Livingstone

Todd I P (1978) Intestinal stomas, Heinemann

Weir J Abrahams P (1978) An atlas of radiological anatomy, Pitman Medical

Articles

Chesmore G (1982) Urology, Clinical forum, Nursing Mirror 155 (16) : supplt

Davies J G (1981) Urinary tract emergencies, British Medical Journal 282 (6258): 111-113

Iveson-Iveson J (1980) The urinary system, multiple choice questions, Nursing Mirror 150 (9): 24

Jones N (1977) Diseases of the urinary system, common urinary symptoms, British Medical Journal 2 (6090): 818—819

Riddle P R (1981) Urothelial tumours, Hospital Update 7 (9): 909-920

Roberts A (1977) Urine — 1, body fluids, Nursing Times : supplt

Roberts A (1978) Urine — 2, body fluids, Nursing Times 74 (3): supplt

Roberts A Systems of Life no. 23, U.G. 1 kidney, Nursing Times

Roberts A Systems of Life no. 24, U.G. 2 Ureters and bladder, Nursing Times

(1977) The symposium on urological problems, Practitioner 218 (1303): 59-96

(1979) The symposium on genitourinary problems, Practitioner 223 (1335): 305-346

(1982) The symposium on genitourinary disorders, Practitioner 226 (1373): 1835-1916

(1980) Urinary nursing, Community Outlook, Nursing Times 76 (15): supplt

Index